Amy A. Eyler, PhD
Editor

Environmental, Policy, and Cultural Factors Related to Physical Activity in a Diverse Sample of Women: The Women's Cardiovascular Health Network Project

Environmental, Policy, and Cultural Factors Related to Physical Activity in a Diverse Sample of Women: The Women's Cardiovascular Health Network Project has been co-published simultaneously as *Women & Health*, Volume 36, Number 2 2002.

"This book contains chapters written by the leading scholars interested in physical activity barriers and facilitators specific to women. The interesting and unique thing about the book is that it examines barriers and facilitators of physical activity from environmental, policy, and cultural perspectives. To my knowledge, no prior book has effectively synthesized this information for a variety of ethnic groups. This book brilliantly achieves that end result.

One strength of the book is that it takes practical, first-person information from informants on barriers to and facilitators of physical activity and makes recommendations for designing more effective interventions. The use of first-person quotes throughout the book effectively reinforces theoretical concpets presented. Another strength of the book is the snythesis of information across cultures. Although some barriers and facilitators differ across cultures, many are similar. Denoting the differences and similiarities between cultures should help intervention specialists design low-cost, effective physical activity interventions.

This book is a 'must-read' for anyone interested in designing, implementing, and evaluating physical activity interventions for underserved–and typically inactive–women. Other individuals who might be interested in this book include those who conduct qualitative research and/or those interested in reading more about one of the most important large-scale national studies of women in this decade. I plan to use this book for my graduate course in 'Physical Activity Interventions.' It effectively synthesizes current information and presents a number of areas ripe for future exploration."

Lynda Ransdell, PhD, FACSM
Assistant Professor
of Exercise & Sport Science
University of Utah
Salt Lake City, UT

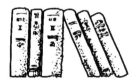

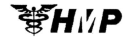

The Haworth Medical Press
An Imprint of The Haworth Press, Inc.

Environmental, Policy, and Cultural Factors Related to Physical Activity in a Diverse Sample of Women: The Women's Cardiovascular Health Network Project

Environmental, Policy, and Cultural Factors Related to Physical Activity in a Diverse Sample of Women: The Women's Cardiovascular Health Network Project has been co-published simultaneously as *Women & Health*, Volume 36, Number 2 2002.

The *Women & Health* Monographic "Separates"

Below is a list of "separates," which in serials librarianship means a special issue simultaneously published as a special journal issue or double-issue *and* as a "separate" hardbound monograph. (This is a format which we also call a "DocuSerial.")

"Separates" are published because specialized libraries or professionals may wish to purchase a specific thematic issue by itself in a format which can be separately cataloged and shelved, as opposed to purchasing the journal on an on-going basis. Faculty members may also more easily consider a "separate" for classroom adoption.

"Separates" are carefully classified separately with the major book jobbers so that the journal tie-in can be noted on new book order slips to avoid duplicate purchasing.

You may wish to visit Haworth's website at . . .

http://www.HaworthPress.com

. . . to search our online catalog for complete tables of contents of these separates and related publications.

You may also call 1-800-HAWORTH (outside US/Canada: 607-722-5857), or Fax: 1-800-895-0582 (outside US/Canada: 607-771-0012), or e-mail at:

getinfo@haworthpressinc.com

Environmental, Policy, and Cultural Factors Related to Physical Activity in a Diverse Sample of Women: The Women's Cardiovascular Health Network Project, edited by Amy A. Eyler, PhD (Vol. 36, No. 2, 2002). *"INTERESTING AND UNIQUE. . . . A MUST-READ for anyone interested in designing, implementing, and evaluating physical activity interventions for underserved–and typically inactive–women." (Lynda Randsell, PhD, FACSM, Assistant Professor of Exercise & Sport Science, University of Utah-Salt Lake City)*

Women's Health in Mainland Southeast Asia, edited by Andrea Whittaker, PhD (Vol. 35, No. 4, 2002). *Shows how war, military regimes, industrialization, urbanization, and social upheaval have all affected the choices Southeast Asian women make about their health and health care.*

Domestic Violence and Health Care: Policies and Prevention, edited by Carolina Reyes, MD, William J. Rudman, PhD, and Calvin R. Hewitt, MBA (Vol. 35, No. 2/3, 2002). *Examines the role of health care in the struggle to combat domestic violence.*

Women's Work, Health and Quality of Life, edited by Afaf Ibrahim Meleis, PhD, FAAN (Vol. 33, No. 1/2, 2001). *"A FINE COLLECTION. . . . A useful supplement for courses on women and health. It is particularly helpful to have a collection that reports research on women in different countries. . . . Describes role overload, role strain, and stress that occurs when immigrants try to adjust to a new culture." (Eleanor Krassen Covan, PhD, Professor of Sociology, Director of Gerontology, University of North Carolina, Wilmington)*

Welfare, Work and Well-Being, edited by Mary Clare Lennon, PhD, MS (Vol. 32, No. 1/2 & No. 3, 2001). *Examines the relationship between social roles, economic circumstances, material hardship, and child well-being among low-income women.*

Australian Women's Health: Innovations in Social Science and Community Research, edited by Lenore Manderson, PhD (Vol. 28, No. 1, 1998). *Reflects a wider approach to women's health, which moves from maternity and fertility issues to question the impact of gender on all aspects of the disease experience.*

Women, Drug Use and HIV Infection, edited by Sally J. Stevens, PhD, Stephanie Tortu, PhD, and Susan L. Coyle, PhD (Vol. 27, No. 1/2, 1998). *"A much-needed resource of critical information about the largest initiative to date designed to prevent HIV among drug users and their sexual partners." (Robert E. Booth, PhD, Associate Professor of Psychiatry, University of Colorado School of Medicine, Denver)*

Women in the Later Years: Health, Social, and Cultural Perspectives, edited by Lois Grau, PhD, RN, in collaboration with Ida Susser, PhD (Vol. 14, No. 3/4, 1989). *"An excellent overview of the pertinent social, political, and personal issues of this long-ignored group." (News for Women in Psychiatry)*

Government Policy and Women's Health Care: The Swedish Alternative, edited by Gunnela Westlander, PhD, and Jeanne Mager Stellman, PhD (Vol. 13, No. 3/4, 1988). *"An illuminating, comprehensive overview of Swedish women's health and their productive and reproductive roles." (Freda L. Paltiel, Senior Advisor, Status of Women, Health and Welfare Canada, Ottawa, Ontario, Canada)*

Embryos, Ethics, and Women's Rights: Exploring the New Reproductive Technologies, edited by Elaine Hoffman Baruch, Amadeo F. D'Adamo, Jr., and Joni Seager (Vol. 13, No. 1/2, 1988). *"Groundbreaking . . . Reveals the myriad of perspectives from which the new technologies can be regarded. Particularly thought-provoking are discussions that link surrogacy to economic and class issues." (Publishers Weekly)*

Women, Health, and Poverty (also published as Dealing with the Health Needs of Women in Poverty), edited by Cesar A. Perales and Lauren S. Young, EdD (Vol. 12, No. 3/4, 1988). *"Succeeds in alerting readers to many important issues. . . Should be useful to public policymakers, researchers, and others interested in understanding the health problems of poor women." (Contemporary Psychology)*

Women and Cancer, edited by Steven D. Stellman, PhD (Vol. 11, No. 3/4, 1987). *"The contributors succeed in increasing the reader's awareness of cancer in women and in stimulating thought processes in reference to the need for further research." (Oncology Nursing Forum)*

Health Needs of Women as They Age, edited by Sharon Golub, PhD, and Rita Jackaway Freedman, PhD (Vol. 10, No. 2/3, 1985). *"The contributors distill a great deal of general information on aging into an easily readable and understandable format . . . A useful primer." (The New England Journal of Medicine)*

Health Care of the Female Adolescent, edited by Sharon Golub, PhD (Vol. 9, No. 2/3, 1985). *"An excellent collection of well-written and carefully selected articles designed to provide up-to-date information about the health problems of adolescent girls." (Journal of the American Medical Women's Association)*

Lifting the Curse of Menstruation: A Feminist Appraisal of the Influence of Menstruation on Women's Lives, edited by Sharon Golub, PhD (Vol. 8, No. 2/3, 1983). *"Crammed with information and well-documented. Written in a professional style, each chapter is followed by extensive lists of notes and references." (Journal of Sex Education and Therapy)*

Obstetrical Intervention and Technology in the 1980s, edited by Diony Young, BA (Vol. 7, No. 3/4, 1983). *"Every family physician and obstetrician in North America should read this book." (Canadian Family Physician)*

Environmental, Policy, and Cultural Factors Related to Physical Activity in a Diverse Sample of Women: The Women's Cardiovascular Health Network Project

Amy A. Eyler, PhD
Editor

Environmental, Policy, and Cultural Factors Related to Physical Activity in a Diverse Sample of Women: The Women's Cardiovascular Health Network Project has been co-published simultaneously as *Women & Health*, Volume 36, Number 2 2002.

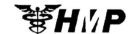

The Haworth Medical Press
An Imprint of
The Haworth Press, Inc.
New York • London • Oxford

Published by

The Haworth Medical Press®, 10 Alice Street, Binghamton, NY 13904-1580 USA

The Haworth Medical Press® is an imprint of The Haworth Press, Inc., 10 Alice Street, Binghamton, NY 13904-1580 USA.

Environmental, Policy, and Cultural Factors Related to Physical Activity in a Diverse Sample of Women: The Women's Cardiovascular Health Network Project has been co-published simultaneously as *Women & Health*, Volume 36, Number 2 2002.

Cover design by Lora Wiggins

Library of Congress Cataloging-in-Publication Data

Environmental, policy, and cultural factors related to physical activity in a diverse sample of women : the Women's Cardiovascular Health Network project / Amy A. Eyler, editor.
     p. ; cm.
    "Co-published simultaneously as Women & health, Volume 36, Number 2, 2002."
    Includes bibliographical references and index.
    ISBN 0-7890-2000-9 (hard. : alk. paper) – ISBN 0-7890-2001-7 (pbk. : alk. paper)
    1. Heart diseases in women–Risk factors. 2. Heart diseases in women–Prevention. 3. Health behavior. 4. Social medicine.
    [DNLM: 1. Women's Cardiovascular Health Network. 2. Women's Health–United States. 3. Cardiovascular Diseases–ethnology–United States. 4. Cultural Diversity–United States. 5. Exercise–United States. 6. Social Environment–United States. 7. Socioeconomic Factors–United States. WA 309 E61 2002] I. Eyler, Amy A.
RA645.C34 E55 2002
616.1′2′0082–dc21
                                             2002012212

Indexing, Abstracting & Website/Internet Coverage

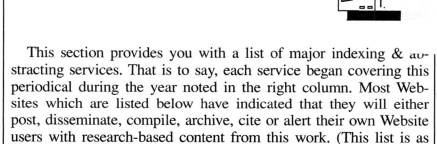

This section provides you with a list of major indexing & abstracting services. That is to say, each service began covering this periodical during the year noted in the right column. Most Websites which are listed below have indicated that they will either post, disseminate, compile, archive, cite or alert their own Website users with research-based content from this work. (This list is as current as the copyright date of this publication.)

Abstracting, Website/Indexing Coverage . . . . Year When Coverage Began

- *Abstracts in Anthropology* **1991**
- *Abstracts in Social Gerontology: Current Literature on Aging* **1991**
- *Academic Abstracts/CD-ROM* **1992**
- *Academic ASAP <www.galegroup.com>* **1988**
- *Academic Search: database of 2,000 selected academic serials, updated monthly: EBSCO Publishing* **1995**
- *Academic Search Elite (EBSCO)* **1993**
- *Behavioral Medicine Abstracts* **1996**
- *Biology Digest (in print & online)* **1991**
- *Cambridge Scientific Abstracts (Health & Safety Science Abstracts/Risk Abstracts) <www.csa.com>* **2001**
- *CINAHL (Cumulative Index to Nursing & Allied Health Literature) <www.cinahl.com>* **1985**
- *CNPIEC Reference Guide: Chinese National Directory of Foreign Periodicals* **1995**
- *Combined Health Information Database (CHID)* **1994**
- *Contemporary Women's Issues* **1998**
- *Criminal Justice Abstracts* **1990**
- *Current Contents/Social & Behavioral Sciences <www.isinet.com>* **1995**

(continued)

(continued)

(continued)

*Special Bibliographic Notes related to special journal issues
(separates) and indexing/abstracting:*

- indexing/abstracting services in this list will also cover material in any "separate" that is co-published simultaneously with Haworth's special thematic journal issue or DocuSerial. Indexing/abstracting usually covers material at the article/chapter level.
- monographic co-editions are intended for either non-subscribers or libraries which intend to purchase a second copy for their circulating collections.
- monographic co-editions are reported to all jobbers/wholesalers/approval plans. The source journal is listed as the "series" to assist the prevention of duplicate purchasing in the same manner utilized for books-in-series.
- to facilitate user/access services all indexing/abstracting services are encouraged to utilize the co-indexing entry note indicated at the bottom of the first page of each article/chapter/contribution.
- this is intended to assist a library user of any reference tool (whether print, electronic, online, or CD-ROM) to locate the monographic version if the library has purchased this version but not a subscription to the source journal.
- individual articles/chapters in any Haworth publication are also available through the Haworth Document Delivery Service (HDDS).

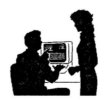

Environmental, Policy, and Cultural Factors Related to Physical Activity in a Diverse Sample of Women: The Women's Cardiovascular Health Network Project

CONTENTS

ABOUT THE EDITOR

Amy A. Eyler, PhD, is Assistant Professor at the St. Louis University School of Public Health. Her research focuses on women and cardiovascular health, particularly on women and physical activity. She has been a member of the Women's Cardiovascular Health Network since 1998 and is currently coordinator of a multi-site research study on the barriers to physical activity among women. She has published extensively on this topic, and one article, for the *Journal of Health Education and Behavior*, "Physical Activity and Minority Women: A Qualitative Study" won Sage Publications' Article of the Year Award in 1998.

Foreword:
Understanding Environmental Influences
on Women's Physical Activity Patterns

With the establishment of the importance of regular physical activity to the health and functioning of the American population throughout the lifespan, an increasing emphasis has been placed on better understanding the factors influencing physical activity levels (U.S. Department of Health and Human Services, 1996). Traditionally, this emphasis has been limited primarily to studying the personal factors (i.e., demographic, cognitive, behavioral, emotional) that may influence people's decisions to become or remain physically active. Indeed, such investigations have yielded a plethora of individual-level variables that appear to influence physical activity participation (King et al., 1992). Yet, it has become increasingly clear that such factors alone cannot account for the substantial prevalence of inactivity in this country. In response to this observation, an emerging interest has developed in exploring broader-level environmental and policy influences on physical activity, in this as well as other industrialized nations (King, 2000; Sallis, Bauman, & Pratt, 1998). Such interests have occurred, in particular, for those population segments reporting especially low physical activity levels–among them, ethnic minority groups and women (Taylor, Baranowski, & Young, 1998; U.S. Department of Health and Human Services, 1996).

The current collection of articles represents ground breaking work in the effort to better understand the role that environmental and policy factors may play in influencing physical activity in several notably understudied target groups of women, including ethnic minority and rural women. Through the application of a standard set of qualitative procedures, these articles shed light on

[Haworth co-indexing entry note]: "Foreword: Understanding Environmental Influences on Women's Physical Activity Patterns." King, Abby C. Co-published simultaneously in *Women & Health* (The Haworth Medical Press, an imprint of The Haworth Press, Inc.) Vol. 36, No. 2, 2002, pp. xv-xviii; and: *Environmental, Policy, and Cultural Factors Related to Physical Activity in a Diverse Sample of Women: The Women's Cardiovascular Health Network Project* (ed: Amy A. Eyler) The Haworth Medical Press, an imprint of The Haworth Press, Inc., 2002, pp. xv-xviii. Single or multiple copies of this article are available for a fee from The Haworth Document Delivery Service [1-800-HAWORTH, 9:00 a.m. - 5:00 p.m. (EST). E-mail address: getinfo@haworthpressinc.com].

xv

a number of the environmental, social, and cultural constraints to a physically active lifestyle facing both urban and non-urban women in this country.

While the samples of underactive women are drawn from diverse regions of the country, and apply a range of different recruitment strategies, the similarities in perceived environmental barriers to becoming physically active are striking. Among such frequently reported barriers were neighborhood threats (e.g., unleashed or stray dogs), lack of positive role models and social or cultural support for physical activity, and, most prominently, a dedication to family and caregiving responsibilities that presented substantial time and logistical barriers to being physically active.

The articles also raised additional questions that merit further exploration using such qualitative methods. These included the reported lack of age-related differences in perceptions and experiences in most of the focus groups that were conducted. While this result may indeed be accurate, it is also possible that the small numbers of women representing any portion of the age range being targeted (20 to 50 years) made it less likely that clear age-related differences would emerge. A more thorough exploration of age-related factors is recommended, particularly with respect to including older (over age 50) age groups of women (who, in fact, represent the most inactive segment of women in the U.S.) (King, Rejeski, & Buchner, 1998; U.S. Department of Health and Human Services, 1996).

A second issue that emerged from the series of focus groups concerned the ambiguous nature of the terms 'physical activity' and 'exercise' for many women. Differences in meaning and connotations surrounding these terms have been underscored by other researchers targeting women (Masse et al., 1998). Clearly, until we gain a better perspective on how best to define and 'capture' the different domains of health-promoting physical activities in a manner that makes sense to women of different backgrounds and cultures, investigations in this area will be hampered.

Although the current series of articles represents among the most diverse array of women that have been studied in this field to date, the lack of focus groups specifically targeting Asian women was notable. A previous qualitative investigation that included Filipino and Chinese women over 40 years of age reported, similar to the current articles, lack of time due to caregiving responsibilities, as well as health concerns and lack of motivation to be physically active during leisure time, as potentially important barriers to becoming more regularly physically active among Asian women (Eyler et al., 1998). Given the fact that Asians are, along with Latinos, the fastest-growing ethnic minority group in the United States (Lin-Fu, 1993; U.S. Bureau of the Census, 1993), and have to date been minimally studied in the physical activity arena (Lew et al., 1999; Taylor et al., 1998), this important ethnic group should be included in future studies.

From the different focus groups, an array of potentially useful environmental and policy-related intervention strategies emerged. Increasing access to appropriate community-based physical activity settings and facilities was frequently suggested. Making such facilities more available to women in these communities may indeed set the stage for increased activity. It is important to note, however, that in several community and worksite studies of women in which access to convenient and inexpensive exercise facilities (including on-site child care, in some cases) was systematically increased, physical activity levels among participants remained surprisingly unaffected (and low) (French, Jeffery, & Oliphant, 1994). Such studies underscore one of the limitations of focus groups and similar self-report methods, i.e., individuals' perceptions of what may help or hinder a particular behavior may, in fact, be erroneous. It is therefore imperative that the hypotheses generated by such qualitative methods be submitted to more systematic and rigorous evaluation prior to their being acted upon. Such quantitative investigations can help to shed light on not only the utility and relevance of individuals' personal observations in these arenas, but, also, the circumstances under which such environmental and cultural factors may be most likely to operate. For example, in a recently completed study of rural communities, increasing facility access through the presence of community walking trails *was* linked to reported increases in walking among at least some groups of community women (Brownson et al., 2000).

Given the apparent complexity of factors spanning personal, environmental, cultural, and policy levels of analysis, and the importance of family in the lives of many women, it has become clear that physical activity interventions will likely need to be both multi-level and multi-generational in focus. In addition, they will need to be tailored to the circumstances of specific locales and cultures, if we are to have a chance at stemming the tide of inactivity facing current as well as future generations of women. The current articles represent an important early step in that endeavor.

Abby C. King, PhD
Division of Epidemiology
Department of Health Research & Policy
Stanford Center for Research in Disease Prevention
Department of Medicine
Stanford University School of Medicine
730 Welch Road, Suite B
Palo Alto, CA 94304-1583
E-mail: king@stanford.edu

REFERENCES

Brownson, R. C., Housemann, R. A., Brown, D. R., Jackson-Thompson, J., King, A. C., Malone, B. R., & Sallis, J. F. (2000). Promoting physical activity in rural communities: Walking trail access, use, and effects. *American Journal of Preventive Medicine, 18*, 235-241.

Eyler, A. A., Baker, E., Cromer, L., King, A. C., Brownson, R. C., & Donatelle, R. J. (1998). Physical activity and minority women: A qualitative study. *Health Education and Behavior, 25*, 640-652.

French, S. A., Jeffery, R. W., & Oliphant, J. A. (1994). Facility access and self-reward as methods to promote physical activity among healthy sedentary adults. *American Journal of Health Promotion, 8*, 257-262.

King, A. C. (2000). Environmental and policy approaches to the promotion of physical activity. In J. M. Rippe (Ed.), *Lifestyle medicine* (pp. 1295-1308). Norwalk, CT: Blackwell Science, Inc.

King, A. C., Blair, S. N., Bild, D. E., Dishman, R. K., Dubbert, P. M., Marcus, B. H., Oldridge, N. B., Paffenbarger Jr., R. S., Powell, K. E., & Yeager, K. K. (1992). Determinants of physical activity and interventions in adults. *Medicine and Science in Sports and Exercise, 24 (supplement 6)*, S221-S236.

King, A. C., Rejeski, W. J., & Buchner, D. M. (1998). Physical activity interventions targeting older adults: A critical review and recommendations. *American Journal of Preventive Medicine, 15*, 316-333.

Lew, R., Chau, J., Woo, J. M., Nguyen, K. D., Okahara, L., Min, K. J., & Lee, D. (1999). Annual walkathons as a community education strategy for the Asian American/Pacific Islander populations in Alameda County, California. *Journal of Health Education, 30 (March/April supplement) (2)*, S25-S30.

Lin-Fu, J. S. (1993). Asian and Pacific Islander Americans: An overview of demographic characteristics and health care issues. *Asian American and Pacific Islander Journal of Health, 1*, 20-34.

Masse, L. C., Ainsworth, B. E., Tortolero, S., Levin, S., Fulton, J. E., Henderson, K. A., & Mayo, K. (1998). Measuring physical activity in midlife, older, and minority women: issues from an expert panel. *Journal of Women's Health, 7*, 57-67.

Sallis, J. F., Bauman, A., & Pratt, M. (1998). Environmental and policy interventions to promote physical activity. *American Journal of Preventive Medicine, 15*, 379-397.

Taylor, W. C., Baranowski, T., & Young, D. R. (1998). Physical activity interventions in low-income, ethnic minority, and populations with disability. *American Journal of Preventive Medicine, 15*, 334-343.

U.S. Bureau of the Census. (1993). *We the Americans: Asians*. Washington, DC: U.S. Government Printing Office.

U.S. Department of Health and Human Services. (1996). *Physical activity and health: A report of the Surgeon General*. Atlanta, GA: U.S. Department of Health and Human Services, Centers for Disease Control and Prevention, National Center for Chronic Disease Prevention and Health Promotion.

Environmental, Policy, and Cultural Factors Related to Physical Activity in a Diverse Sample of Women: The Women's Cardiovascular Health Network Project– Introduction and Methodology

Amy A. Eyler, PhD
Joshua R. Vest, MPH
Bonnie Sanderson, PhD
JoEllen Wilbur, PhD

Dyann Matson-Koffman, PhD
Kelly R. Evenson, PhD
Janice L. Thompson, PhD
Sara Wilcox, PhD

Deborah Rohm Young, PhD

Amy A. Eyler and Joshua R. Vest are affiliated with Saint Louis University, School of Public Health, Prevention Research Center, St. Louis, MO 63104. Dyann Matson-Koffman is affiliated with the Cardiovascular Health Branch, Division of Adult and Community Health, National Center for Chronic Disease Prevention and Health Promotion, CDC, Atlanta, GA 30341-3724. Kelly R. Evenson is affiliated with the University of North Carolina-Chapel Hill, School of Public Health, Department of Epidemiology, Chapel Hill, NC 27514. Bonnie Sanderson is affiliated with the University of Alabama, Birmingham, AL 35294. Janice L. Thompson is affiliated with the Department of Pediatrics, Center for Health Promotion & Disease Prevention, University of New Mexico Sciences Center, Albuquerque, NM 87131. JoEllen Wilbur is affiliated with the University of Illinois at Chicago, Department of Public Health, Mental Health, and Administrative Nursing, College of Nursing, Chicago, IL 60612-7350. Sara Wilcox is affiliated with the Department of Exercise Science, Norman J. Arnold School of Public Health, University of South Carolina, Columbia, SC 29208. Deborah Rohm Young is affiliated with Johns Hopkins University, Welch Center for Prevention, Epidemiology, and Clinical Research, Baltimore, MD 21205.

Address correspondence to: Amy A. Eyler, PhD, Saint Louis University, School of Public Health, Prevention Research Center, 3545 Lafayette Avenue, St. Louis, MO 63104 (E-mail: eyleras@accessus.net).

[Haworth co-indexing entry note]: "Environmental, Policy, and Cultural Factors Related to Physical Activity in a Diverse Sample of Women: The Women's Cardiovascular Health Network Project–Introduction and Methodology." Eyler, Amy A. et al. Co-published simultaneously in *Women & Health* (The Haworth Medical Press, an imprint of The Haworth Press, Inc.) Vol. 36, No. 2, 2002, pp. 1-15; and: *Environmental, Policy, and Cultural Factors Related to Physical Activity in a Diverse Sample of Women: The Women's Cardiovascular Health Network Project* (ed: Amy A. Eyler) The Haworth Medical Press, an imprint of The Haworth Press, Inc., 2002, pp. 1-15. Single or multiple copies of this article are available for a fee from The Haworth Document Delivery Service [1-800-HAWORTH, 9:00 a.m. - 5:00 p.m. (EST). E-mail address: getinfo@haworthpressinc.com].

SUMMARY. Ethnic minority and low-income populations have some of the highest rates of cardiovascular disease (CVD) and the highest rates of physical inactivity, an independent risk factor for CVD. Ethnic minority and low-income women are especially at risk. Because programs designed to increase physical activity have the potential to reduce CVD rates in specific populations, research in this area is expanding. As part of the Women's Cardiovascular Health Network funded by the Centers for Disease Control and Prevention, the goal of this multi-site project is to identify factors, particularly environmental, policy, and cultural factors, that may influence physical activity among ethnic minority and low-income women ages 20-50 years. To achieve this goal, 42 focus groups were conducted in various locations throughout the United States with African American, American Indian, Latina and White women. Groups represented both urban and rural living environments. This article explains the basis for this project and the methodology used. Other articles in this series explain the results from the focus groups in detail. *[Article copies available for a fee from The Haworth Document Delivery Service: 1-800-HAWORTH. E-mail address: <getinfo@ haworthpressinc.com> Website: <http://www.HaworthPress.com> © 2002 by The Haworth Press, Inc. All rights reserved.]*

KEYWORDS. Physical activity, women's health, exercise, determinants

INTRODUCTION AND BACKGROUND

A large body of research has established that regular physical activity reduces the risk of premature death and disability from a variety of health conditions, cardiovascular disease in particular (USDHHS, 1996). Ethnic minority and low income populations, often having the highest rates of cardiovascular disease (CVD), also have the highest rates of physical inactivity, an independent risk factor for this disease (CDC, 1993).

Women report less leisure-time physical activity than men (Jones, 1998). Data from the 1998 Behavioral Risk Factor Surveillance System (BRFSS) indicate that 30% of women report no leisure time physical activity compared with 27% of men (CDC, 2000). Additionally, fewer women meet the recommended amounts of physical activity than men (Macera & Pratt, 2000; CDC, 2001).

Women are not optimally physically active for many reasons. One of the main reasons is lack of time due to caretaking responsibilities (Brownson et al., 2000a; Eyler et al., 1998; King, 1997). Other personal barriers include lack of motivation, poor perceptions of health, and lack of self-efficacy (Eyler et al., 1998; Eyler et al., 2002). Lack of social support also influences the physical activity level of women (CDC, 1998; Eyler, Brownson, Donatelle, Brown, & Sallis, 1999; Verhoef, Love, & Rose, 1992; Yoshida, Allison, & Osborn, 1988). Environmental (e.g., lack of safe places to exercise) and policy (e.g., lack of flex time at work to exercise) barriers also affect physical activity levels in women (Eyler et al., 2002).

The correlates vary by the type of physical activity. Correlates of leisure-time physical activity differ from those of household, caregiving, cultural dancing, and other types of less traditionally studied physical activities. Presence of children and caregiving responsibilities may increase household physical activity, but such responsibilities can hinder sports or exercise (Sternfeld, Ainsworth, & Quesenberry, 1999).

Women of color are less active than White women. Data from the 1994 BRFSS found that 46% of African American women reported no leisure-time physical activity in the past month compared with 30% of White women (Bolen et al., 2000). Several factors identified to explain this include not knowing the importance of exercise (Carter-Nolan, Adams-Campbell, & Williams, 1996), health problems (Broman, 1995), mental fatigue from physically demanding labor (both job and family related), and a need to compensate by resting (Kriska & Rexroad, 1998; Nies, Vollman, & Cook, 1999). Particularly illuminating are findings that minority women do not believe they have leisure time as conventionally defined (Airhihenbuwa, Kumanyika, Agurs, & Lowe, 1995; Yeager, Macera, & Merrit, 1993), and perceive exercising to be an unaffordable indulgence (Kriska & Rexroad, 1998).

Cultural factors may also affect physical activity levels in African American women. Compared with White women, African American women are more satisfied with their weight and, if overweight, are more likely to feel attractive (Flynn & Fitzgibbons, 1998). This cultural difference, however, places African American women at greater risk for obesity and thus makes it less likely that they will lose weight when indicated. In addition, at least one study suggests that African Americans may place higher value on rest than being physically active during leisure time (Airhihenbuwa, Kumanyika, Agurs, & Lowe, 1995). Additional common social and cultural values among African Americans such as kinship, collectivism, the importance of music and religion (Willis, 1992), as well as views of health and wellness (Kumanyika, Wilson, & Guilford-Davenport, 1993), are also likely to significantly impact physical activity behaviors.

Other racial/ethnic groups, although less-studied than African American or White women, also demonstrate higher rates of physical inactivity and less leisure-time physical activity. For example, the BRFSS found the prevalence of no leisure activity in the past month was 39% for Hispanic women but 28% for White women (USHSS, 1996). American Indian women also have lower levels of reported physical activity (Welty et al., 1995; Ellis & Campos-Outcalt, 1994; Brownson et al., 2000). Many women in these groups have additional barriers to physical activity including varying levels of acculturation, language barriers, and culturally dictated gender roles.

In addition to gender, living environment and socioeconomic status are shown to be correlates of physical activity. Data from the BRFSS indicate that physical inactivity is highest in rural areas (37%) and lowest in metropolitan areas (27%) (CDC, 1998). Among rural areas, those in the South have the highest rates (44%). In the US Women's Determinants Study (Brownson et al., 2000; Wilcox et al., 2000), a random-digit telephone survey of ethnically diverse women aged 40 years and older, rural women were significantly more likely than urban women to report no participation in exercise, recreational activities, or physical activities.

Because programs designed to increase physical activity have the potential to reduce CVD rates, particularly in underserved groups, research in this area is expanding. Projects in many states have been funded to reduce disparities in CVD through policy and environmental interventions designed to improve physical activity and nutrition behaviors. Unfortunately, although some data identify the association between environmental factors and these behaviors (Bauman & Bellew, 1999), and theory proposes the environment's importance in behavior change (McElroy et al., 1988; Sallis et al., 1998) there is little reported evidence that these types of interventions are effective in changing the targeted behaviors, particularly among ethnic/minority populations.

In 1998, the National Heart, Lung, Blood Institute (NHLBI) Task Force on Behavioral Research in Cardiovascular Disease stated that "Research is needed on the effects of the broader environment on adoption of dietary and physical activity . . . and this knowledge should be used to develop more effective policies and population-based interventions for primary prevention" (NHLBI, 1998). More recently, the Women's Cardiovascular Health Network was funded by the Centers for Disease Control and Prevention (CDC) to identify factors that promote cardiovascular health in women in 1998. This network coordinated an expert panel that evaluated literature on physical activity, nutrition, and smoking cessation interventions for women. A comprehensive review was published (Krummel et al., 2001) and the panel recommended that additional formative and qualitative research be conducted in order to examine the mediating factors that facilitate the role of policy and environmental interventions in influencing physical activity, dietary and tobacco behaviors among women.

Based on these findings, CDC funded this research as a special interest project through the Prevention Research Centers. The Robert Wood Johnson Foundation provided additional funding to expand the number of research sites. The goal of this two-year, multi-site project is to identify factors, particularly cultural, environmental, and policy ones, that are important in influencing physical activity among ethnic/minority and low income women ages 20-50 years. This project was approved by the Institutional Review Board (IRB) of CDC and each university involved. The populations targeted and affiliated universities funded to implement the project are listed in Table 1.

Findings from this research will be used to help State Health Departments and other partners (e.g., community coalitions) to effectively plan, design, and implement culturally appropriate community, policy and environmental interventions for physical activity in ethnic/minority and low socioeconomic populations. The information may also be used to influence policy makers to allocate resources for specific environmental changes and to support physical activity policy.

METHODS

A literature search to identify knowledge and gaps in knowledge about correlates of physical activity in the subgroups of interest (Eyler et al., 2002) permitted the team to create core questions for a qualitative study using focus groups to help identify cultural, environmental, and policy factors as potential barriers or enablers of physical activity. The core questions (without probes), listed in Table 2, were designed to identify important factors that may influence physical activity levels among diverse groups of women. The literature review revealed few relevant correlates, so qualitative research methods were preferred to a quantitative approach.

TABLE 1. Populations Studied and Affiliated Universities

Race/Ethnicity	Living Environment*	University
African American	Urban	• University of Illinois-Chicago • Johns Hopkins University
African American	Rural	• University of Alabama-Birmingham
African American	Metropolitan	• University of South Carolina
American Indian	Rural	• University of New Mexico
Latina	Rural	• University of North Carolina at Chapel Hill
White	Rural	• Saint Louis University

* The living environments were determined by US Census information. Each site was classified according to the rural-urban continuum codes of the Office of Management and Budget. Counties are classified as metro (4 possible subcategories) or non-metro (6 possible subcategories). (US Department of Agriculture, 2000.) Because these definitions changed from the 1990 Census, the USC counties were previously categorized as rural, but now are considered metropolitan.

TABLE 2. Focus Group Questions

*1. *Think about all the ways women your age can be physically active. Name a few.*

*2. *When you think of a physically active (insert racial/ethnic group) woman, what images come to mind?*

*3. *When you think of a physically inactive (insert racial/ethnic group) woman, what images come to mind?*

4. *How does living in your household make a difference in your physical activity level?*

5. *Think about your neighborhood. What is it about your neighborhood that makes it easy or hard for you to be physically active?*

6. *What things at work make it easier/harder for you to be more physically active?*

7. *How does living in your city or town make it easier/harder for you to be more physically active?*

8. *Let's say you are a community leader. You have the power and the resources to make changes. How would you help other women in your community or neighborhood be more physically active?*

9. *Now let's say you are the boss (owner, CEO) of a company. How would you help women in this workplace be more physically active?*

10. *Do you think women with different cultural backgrounds (e.g., African American, Latina, Asian) have different levels of physical activity in their daily lives? If so, Why?*

*Not discussed in this article. Because the amount of information obtained from the focus groups was so great, the research team decided to narrow the scope and focus on environmental, policy and cultural issues.

Focus group leaders for each site were chosen for their connection to the community being studied. Most often, the leader was of the same race/ethnicity as the participants in the group. Each site was responsible for training the leaders and adhering to the moderator's guide developed by the group. In addition to the focus group leader, a note-taker was also present to keep a brief written account of conversation and the non-verbal nuances of the group.

Codes were developed from concepts found in the literature review and in an ecological model proposed by McLeroy and colleagues (McElroy et al., 1988), where health behavior is determined by 5 levels of influence: (1) intrapersonal factors (psychological and biological factors and developmental history), (2) interpersonal processes and primary groups (formal and informal social network and support systems including family, friends, and coworkers), (3) institutional factors (social institutions such as schools, health agencies, and companies), (4) community factors (relationships among organizations, institutions, and informal networks), and (5) public policy (local, state, and national laws and policies). Although this model does not specifically address the role of physical environmental factors in health promotion, physical factors have been seen as critical elements of an ecological model of physical activity (Sallis et al., 1998). Ecological models differ from many other theoretical models in that they emphasize factors outside of the individual that influence behavior. Accordingly, these models can aid in understanding the determinants of physical activity in minority women because they recognize societal, organizational, and other external constraints placed on women that may limit their participation.

Our analysis included the use of "axial coding," a process that identifies ideas and themes and organizes key concepts. One advantage of axial coding is that it stimulates thinking about linkages between concepts, and the connection between a theme and data can be strengthened by multiple instances of empirical evidence (Neuman, 1994). The use of a common, structured coding theme facilitated collaboration between the sites and allowed for better consistency in analysis across sites than traditional open coding.

Because the literature review revealed that more is known about personal barriers to physical activity than environmental barriers, the research team has focused this study on barriers to physical activity with regard to culture, environment, and policy. These terms, and community, can be defined as follows:

Community: a social unit that usually encompasses a geographic region in which residents live and interact socially, such as a political subunit (e.g., a county or town) or a smaller area (e.g., a neighborhood or a housing complex). A community may be a social organization (a formal or informal group of people who share common interests, such as a faith organization). An individual may be a member of several communities or subgroups defined by a variety of factors, such as age, sex, occupation, socioeconomic status, activities, culture, or history (CDC, 2000).

Environment: A community environment encompasses all settings for which policies, social environments and physical space can be manipulated at some level. Examples include retail businesses and public space such as parks, sidewalks, and green ways. Environmental changes would, therefore, be those changes necessary to foster and maintain individual-level behavior change to improve physical activity levels (CDC, 2000).

Policy: Policy refers to a legislative, regulatory, or policy-making action that has potential to affect physical activity. These approaches may be formal legal actions taken by local, state, or federal governments (Sallis et al., 1998). Organizational policies are those that specific organizations, such as schools, worksite, or health care organizations, create in order to define appropriate behavior within the confines of the organization (Schmid et al., 1995).

Culture: Culture refers to attitudes, norms, and values shared by a group that may affect individual behavior. Examples of cultural effects include the kinds of ideas people hold, obligations they feel, or values they espouse that may lead them to behave in the way they do (Adamopoulos & Kashima, 1990).

Six to eight focus groups were conducted at each site, with groups ranging from 2 to 10 participants. Each site attempted to complete three groups with women ages 20-35 years, and three groups with women ages 36-50 years. By dividing the women into two age groups, we hoped to identify potential life-stage differences. The sites used different recruitment methods but the same inclusion criteria for participants. Criteria for inclusion in this study were: age 20-50 years (as stated by the grant from the funding organization), currently not a regular exerciser (defined as moderate intensity exercise at least 3 times a week for at least 20 minutes at a time), being of the race/ethnicity of interest, and residing in the community being studied. To collect basic demographic information, a brief quantitative survey was given to participants after each focus group (see Table 3).

Each focus group's discussion was audiotaped, transcribed verbatim (and translated, if Latina), and then coded. To ensure reliability in coding the transcripts across the research sites, a sample transcript was coded by every member of the research team. The researchers at each university often discussed the code book discrepancies and modified it accordingly. Also, at each site, the transcripts were coded with the consensus of at least two people. Since the populations studied varied by race/ethnicity and living environment, most sites added additional codes tailored to these populations. For example, in the Latina and American Indian groups, unique cultural issues were discussed (e.g., acculturation). Codes that related to culture were added for these groups, but not for the White or African American groups.

The coded transcripts were then analyzed using QSR NUD*IST qualitative software. Each site followed a common outline for analysis. Each site explored themes and issues relevant to their group, in addition to those topics decided a priori.

LIMITATIONS

As with all focus group research, our approach had some limitations. First, generalizability from focus groups is limited and this may be especially true for minority groups that consist of many subcultures. For example, the information gained from a highly acculturated group of Pueblo women sampled by the New Mexico site may not be generalizable to other American Indian

TABLE 3. Demographic Information on Focus Group Participants

	White[1]	African American[2]	African American[3]	African American[4]	African American[5]	Am. Indian[6]	Latina[7]	Total
Number	33	42	61	42	48	30	49	305
Age								
Mean	37.4	31.8	35.6	38.5	36.9	37.4	32.5	35.6
Median	38.0	30.0	37.0	39.0	36.0	37.0	32.0	36.0
Marital status								
% married/unmarried couple	78.8	21.4	32.8	38.1	14.6	43.3	87.8	43.9
% unmarried	21.2	78.6	63.9	61.9	84.5	56.7	8.2	54.8
Education								
% college grad	30.3	0	18.0	23.8	2.1	13.3	10.2	13.4
% some college	36.4	61.9	49.2	57.1	33.3	56.7	16.3	44.5
% HS grad	27.3	21.4	24.6	16.7	31.3	26.7	18.4	23.6
% less than HS	3.0	16.7	8.2	2.4	33.3	3.3	55.1	18.5
Self-reported BMI-kg/m^2 (mean)	27.8	28.8	34.2	29.5	32.4	35.1	29.1	31.3
# of adults in home	2.2	2.3	2.0	2.1	2.4	2.6	2.6	2.3
# of children in home	1.4	1.4	2.1	1.1	2.9	2.2	2.2	1.9
Self-described general health (%)								
Excellent	12.1	12.2	4.9	11.9	10.4	0	0	7.2
Very good	30.3	22.0	24.6	23.8	20.8	10.0	18.4	21.6
Good	48.5	51.2	52.5	52.4	31.3	53.3	38.8	46.2
Fair	9.1	9.8	14.8	11.9	33.3	36.7	28.6	20.3
Poor	0	4.9	3.3	0	4.2	0	0	2.0

TABLE 3 (continued)

	White[1]	African American[2]	African American[3]	African American[4]	African American[5]	Am. Indian[6]	Latina[7]	Total
Employment (%)								
Employed full time	42.4	26.2	49.2	76.2	35.4	66.7	14.3	43.0
Employed part time	18.2	16.7	27.9	2.4	8.3	3.3	10.2	13.4
Self-employed	18.2	7.1	4.9	4.8	8.3	6.7	6.1	7.5
Out of work	3.0	33.3	6.6	0	22.9	10.0	20.4	14.1
Homemaker	15.2	2.4	1.6	4.8	10.4	10.0	46.9	13.1
Student	0	9.5	3.3	2.4	2.1	3.3	0	3.0
Retired	0	0	0	2.4	0	0	0	0.3
Unable to work	3.0	2.4	3.3	2.4	8.3	0	0	3.0
Typical work day (%)								
Mostly sitting/standing	15.2	25.5	19.7	31.0	12.5	6.7	16.3	16.7
1/2 sitting/standing & 1/2 walking	39.4	45.0	34.4	38.1	25.0	40.0	12.2	29.2
Mostly walking	9.1	30.0	21.3	11.9	16.7	6.7	22.4	15.7
1/2 heavy work & 1/2 sitting/standing	9.1	0	1.6	2.4	4.2	13.3	4.1	4.3
1/2 heavy work & 1/2 walking	0	0	1.6	2.4	2.1	3.3	4.1	2.0
Physically demanding	0	0	6.6	2.4	6.3	3.3	0	3.0
Typical non-work day(%)								
Mostly sitting/standing	18.2	36.6	18.0	28.6	29.2	13.3	26.5	24.6
1/2 sitting/standing & 1/2 walking	48.5	34.1	36.1	38.1	25.0	53.3	32.7	36.7
Mostly walking	6.1	12.2	11.5	9.5	18.8	3.3	26.5	13.4
1/2 heavy work & 1/2 sitting/standing	21.2	9.5	14.8	11.9	14.6	16.7	4.1	12.8
1/2 heavy work & 1/2 walking	0	4.8	11.5	4.8	6.3	3.3	4.1	5.6
Physically demanding	0	2.4	4.9	0	4.2	6.7	0	2.6
Days a week do moderate activity	3.6	4.2	2.8	3.4	4.9	4.1	4.4	3.78
Days a week do vigorous activity	0.5	0.3	0.5	0.4	0.4	0.4	0.6	0.46

[1] Rural–Saint Louis University
[2] Metropolitan–University of South Carolina
[3] Rural–University of Alabama-Birmingham
[4] Urban–Johns Hopkins University
[5] Urban–University of Illinois-Chicago
[6] Rural & Urban–University of New Mexico
[7] Rural–University of North Carolina at Chapel Hill

women. Another common limitation of focus group methodology is selection bias; most of the participants thought the location and time were convenient. In contrast, women who met the criteria, but may have had other constraints, such as no transportation or no child care, declined participation.

Since we were limited by the request of the funding agency to study only women aged 20-50, we were unable to research older women and compare the results. Also, our study did not include Asian women. The populations were chosen by the researchers based on local demographics and connection to the community being studied, and the final researchers were chosen by the funding agency. Despite these limitations, focus group methodology remains a viable way to gain information that is not easily obtained through quantitative methods (Krueger, 1994).

Another concern was the discrepancy between the way in which the women reported their physical activity levels in the screening process and in the series of physical activity assessment questions on the demographic survey (Table 3). The exercise screening question, which was answered on the telephone or face-to-face, defined exercise as moderate intensity activities occuring at least 3 times a week for at least 20 minutes at a time, with further explanation by the interviewer if necessary. Using data from this question, all participants were characterized as not regular exercisers. On the demographic survey however, the BRFSS series of questions on physical activity was asked (see Appendix). When physical activity rates were calculated from the BRFSS questions, many of the women were classified as being regularly active. One possible explanation for this discrepancy is the difference in how women perceived physical activity. The screening question was concise and described exercise in a "traditional" sense while the BRFSS assessed accumulated physical activity. Women may have confused "busyness" with physical activity. One conclusion that we can draw is that assessing physical activity in women warrants further exploration.

CONCLUSION

Each research site plans to continue work in the communities where the groups were held. Focus group data will be used to design a structured quantitative instrument to (1) validate the qualitative results in a broader sample of women; (2) determine if factors identified in the focus groups predict physical activity level; and (3) provide information on factors amenable to change and thus potential targets of intervention. Results from the quantitative surveys will be shared with local intervention specialists. They will also be given as recommendations to policy makers to assist them in designing programs and making environmental changes to increase physical activity among these populations.

The following articles describe in detail the results of the focus group research from this project. The final paper summarizes the results and offers conclusions and recommendations.

REFERENCES

Adamopoulos, J. & Kashima, Y. (1999). Introduction: Subjective culture as a research tradition. In: *Social psychology and cultural context.* Thousand Oaks, CA: Sage Publications.

Airhihenbuwa, C.O., Kumanyika, S., Agurs, T.D., & Lowe, A. (1995). Perceptions and beliefs about exercise, rest, and health among African-Americans. *American Journal of Health Promotion, 9*(6), 426-429.

Bauman, A. & Bellew, B. (1999). Environmental and policy approaches to promoting physical activity. In Commonwealth Institute (Ed.) *Health in the Commonwealth.* London: Commonwealth Institute.

Broman, C.L. (1995). Leisure-time physical activity in an African-American population. *Journal of Behavioral Medicine, 18*(4), 341-353.

Brownson, R.C., Eyler, A.A., King, A.C., Brown, D.R., Shyu, Y.L., & Sallis, J.F. (2000). Patterns and correlates of physical activity among US women 40 years and older. *American Journal of Public Health, 90*(2), 264-270.

Carter-Nolan, P.L., Adams-Campbell, L.L., & Williams, J. (1996). Recruitment strategies for black women at risk for noninsulin-dependent diabetes mellitus into exercise protocols: A qualitative assessment. *Journal of The National Medical Association, 88*(9), 558-562.

Centers for Disease Control and Prevention. (1997). Monthly estimates of leisure-time physical activity–United States, 1994. *Morbidity and Mortality Weekly Report, 46*(1), 393-397.

Centers for Disease Control and Prevention. (1993). Physical activity and prevention of coronary heart disease. *Morbidity and Mortality Weekly Report, 42*(35), 669-672.

Centers for Disease Control and Prevention. (1995). Prevalence of recommended levels of physical activity among women–Behavioral Risk Factor Surveillance System, 1992. *Morbidity and Mortality Weekly Report, 44*(06), 105-107.

Centers for Disease Control and Prevention. (1998). Self-reported physical inactivity by degree of urbanization–United States, 1996. *Morbidity and Mortality Weekly Report, 47,* 1097-1100.

Centers for Disease Control and Prevention. (2000). Cardiovascular Health Branch (CVHB) grantee semi-annual report. Atlanta, GA: CDC.

Centers for Disease Control and Prevention. (2001). Behavioral Risk Factor Surveillance System Prevalence Data: 2000. *<http://apps.nccd.cdc.gov>.*

Ellis, J.L. & Campos-Outcalt, D. (1994). Cardiovascular disease risk factors in Native Americans: A literature review. *American Journal of Preventive Medicine, 10*(5), 295-307.

Eyler, A., Baker, E., Cromer, L., King, A., Brownson, R., & Donatelle, R. (1998). Physical activity and minority women: A qualitative study. *Health Ed Behavior, 25*, 640-652.

Eyler, A., Brownson, R., Donatelle, R., Brown, D., & Sallis, J. (1999). Physical activity social support and middle-and older-aged minority women: Results from a US survey. *Social Science and Medicine, 49*(6), 781-789.

Eyler, A., Wilcox, S., Matson-Koffman, D., Evenson, K., Sanderson, B., Thompson, J., Wilbur, J., & Young, D.R. (2002). Determinants of physical activity among women from diverse racial/ethnic groups: A review. *Journal of Women's Health and Gender-Based Medicine, 11*(3), 239-253.

Flynn, K.J., & Fitzgibbon, M. (1998). Body images and obesity risk among black females: A review of the literature. *Annals of Behavioral Medicine, 20*(1), 13-24.

Kriska, A.M., & Rexroad, A.R. (1998). The role of physical activity in minority populations. *Women's Health Issues, 8*(2), 98-103.

King, A. (1997). Intervention strategies and determinants of physical activity and exercise behavior in adult and older adult men and women. *World Review of Nutrition and Dietetics, 82*, 148-158.

Krueger, R.A. (1994) *Focus groups: A practical guide for applied research (2nd ed)*. Thousand Oaks, CA: Sage Publications.

Krummel, D.A., Koffman, D.M., Bronner, Y., Davis, J., Greenlund, K., Tessaro, I., Upson, D., & Wilbur, J. (2001). Cardiovascular health interventions in women: What works? *Journal of Women's Health and Gender-Based Medicine, 10*(2), 117-136.

Kumanyika, S., Wilson, J.F., & Guilford-Davenport, M. (1993). Weight-related attitudes and behaviors of black women. *Journal of the American Dietetic Association, 93*, 416-422.

Macera, C.A., & Pratt, M. (2000). Public health surveillance and physical activity. *Research Quarterly for Exercise and Sport, 71*(2), 97-103.

McLeroy, K., Bibeau, D., Steckler, A., & Glanz, K. (1988). An ecological perspective on health promotion programs. *Health Education Quarterly, 15*, 351-377.

Neuman, W.L. (1994). *Social research methods qualitative and quantitative approaches* (2nd Ed), (p. 408). Allyn and Bacon, Boston, MA.

Nies, M.A., Vollman, M., & Cook, T. (1999). African American women's experiences with physical activity in their daily lives. *Public Health Nursing, 16*(1), 23-31.

Sallis, J.F., Bauman, A., & Pratt, M. (1998). Environmental and policy interventions to promote physical activity. *American Journal of Preventive Medicine, 15*(4), 379-397.

Schmid, T.L., Pratt, M., & Howze, E. (1995). Policy as intervention: environmental and policy approaches to the prevention of cardiovascular disease. *American Journal of Public Health, 85*(9), 1207-1211.

Sternfeld, B., Ainsworth, BE., & Quesenberry, C.P. (1999). Physical activity patterns in a diverse population of women. *Preventive Medicine, 28*(13), 313-323.

U.S. Department of Health and Human Services. (1998). *National Heart, Lung, Blood Institute Report of the Taskforce on Behavioral Research in Cardiovascular, Lung, and Blood Health Diseases*. Atlanta, GA: Public Health Service.

U.S. Department of Health and Human Services. (1996). *Physical Activity and Health: A report of the Surgeon General*. Atlanta, GA: US Department of Health and Human Services, Centers for Disease Control and Prevention, National Center for Chronic Disease Prevention and Health Promotion.

U.S. Department of Agriculture. (2000). *<http://www.ers.usda.gov/briefing/rurality/ RuralUrbCon/>*.

Verhoef, M., Love, E., & Rose, M. (1992). Women's social roles and their exercise participation. *Women and Health, 19*(4), 15-28.

Welty, T.K., Lee, E.T., Yeh, J., Cowan, L.D., Go, O., Fabsitz, R.R., Le, N.A., Oopik, A.J., Robbins, D.C., & Howard, B.V. (1995). Cardiovascular disease risk factors among American Indians: The Strong Heart Study. *American Journal of Epidemiology, 142*(3), 269-287.

Wilcox, S., Castro, C., King, A.C., Housemann, R., Brownson, R.C. (2000). Determinants of leisure time physical activity in rural compared with urban older and ethnically diverse women in the United States. *J Epidemiology Community Health*, Sep, *54*(9), 667-672.

Willis, W. (1992). Families with African American roots. In E.W. Lynch & M.J. Hanson (Eds.), *Developing cross-cultural competence. A guide for working with young children and their families* (pp. 121-150). Baltimore: Paul H. Brookes.

Yoshida, K., Allison, K., & Osborn, R. (1988). Social factors influencing perceived barriers to physical activity among women. *Canadian Journal of Public Health, 79*, 104-108.

APPENDIX

Physical activity questions used in brief survey of demographic information. (Source: Behavioral Risk Factor Surveillance System Survey)

In a typical week, do you do moderate activities for at least 10 minutes at a time, such as brisk walking, bicycling, vacuuming, gardening, or anything else that causes some increase in breathing or heart rate?

    ☐ Yes: Days per week _____
    ☐ No

On days when you do moderate activities for at least 10 minutes at a time, how much total time do you spend doing these activities?

    Hours/minutes per day _____

In a typical week, do you do vigorous activities for at least 10 minutes at a time, such as running, aerobics, heavy yard work, or anything else that causes large increases in breathing or heart rate?

    ☐ Yes: Days per week _____
    ☐ No

On days when you do vigorous activities for at least 10 minutes at a time, how much total time do you spend doing these activities?

    Hours/minutes per day _____

Environmental, Policy, and Cultural Factors Related to Physical Activity in Urban, African American Women

JoEllen Wilbur, PhD, RN, CS, FAAN
Peggy Chandler, PhD
Barbara Dancy, PhD, RN
JiWon Choi, MS, RN
Donna Plonczynski, MS, CNP

SUMMARY. This study was part of a multi-site project carried out with seven universities throughout the United States to identify cultural, environmental, and policy determinants of physical activity in ethnic minority women aged 20 to 50 years. Following an extensive literature review, nine core research questions were created to examine potential barriers to physical activity as well as enabling factors. Methods and findings presented are from six focus groups of low-income, urban African American women. These focus groups were held at each of two health centers serving communities in Chicago, Illinois, that are predominantly African American and low income and have households usually headed

---

JoEllen Wilbur is Professor, Peggy Chandler is Research Assistant Professor, Barbara Dancy is Associate Professor, and JiWon Choi and Donna Plonczynski are Doctoral Students, University of Illinois at Chicago, College of Nursing.

Address correspondence to: JoEllen Wilbur, Professor, University of Illinois at Chicago, College of Nursing, 845 South Damen, Chicago, IL 60612 (E-mail: Jwilbur@ UIC.edu).

Funding: SIP 5-99 from the Centers for Disease Control and Prevention.

[Haworth co-indexing entry note]: "Environmental, Policy, and Cultural Factors Related to Physical Activity in Urban, African American Women." Wilbur, JoEllen et al. Co-published simultaneously in *Women & Health* (The Haworth Medical Press, an imprint of The Haworth Press, Inc.) Vol. 36, No. 2, 2002, pp. 17-28; and: *Environmental, Policy, and Cultural Factors Related to Physical Activity in a Diverse Sample of Women: The Women's Cardiovascular Health Network Project* (ed: Amy A. Eyler) The Haworth Medical Press, an imprint of The Haworth Press, Inc., 2002, pp. 17-28. Single or multiple copies of this article are available for a fee from The Haworth Document Delivery Service [1-800-HAWORTH, 9:00 a.m. - 5:00 p.m. (EST). E-mail address: getinfo@haworthpressinc.com].

by women. Forty-eight women participated, with 5 to 11 in each group. Most (85%) were unmarried, 40% had less than a high school education, and 33% were neither employed nor attending school. Findings reflected the influence of a culture of poverty and the importance of environmental safety and community support. The findings will be used to inform the development of community-based exercise interventions and policies that are culturally and socially sensitive to the needs of low-income, urban African American women. *[Article copies available for a fee from The Haworth Document Delivery Service: 1-800-HAWORTH. E-mail address: <getinfo@haworthpressinc.com> Website: <http://www.HaworthPress.com> © 2002 by The Haworth Press, Inc. All rights reserved.]*

KEYWORDS. African American, low income, exercise, physical actvity

PURPOSE

African American women frequently have major risk factors for cardiovascular disease (CVD), including obesity, high blood pressure, and diabetes (NHLB, 1998; AHA, 2001). This excessive burden has far-reaching effects on the family, because African American women are relied on as support networks and as caregiving grandparents (Barker et al., 1998).

Both being physically active in daily routines and exercising regularly show strong evidence of preventing, postponing, or reducing the impact of CVD. Self-report data from the 1992 National Behavioral Risk Factor Surveillance System, however, found African American women to be more likely than white women to have no leisure-time physical activity in the past month (43.6% vs. 27.6%), and physical inactivity was higher among women without a high school education than among college-educated women (47.4% vs. 22.3%) (BRFSS, 1995).

Despite the prevalent risk factors for CVD and related high mortality among African American women, there have been few efforts to encourage health promotion and disease prevention behaviors in this group. A recent review (Krummel et al., 2001) of 19 studies that used behavioral strategies to increase physical activity revealed only three (Cardinal & Sachs, 1996; Chen et al., 1998; Lasco et al., 1989) that addressed African American women, only one of which targeted low-income women (Lasco et al., 1989).

The record for CVD risk factors and the low activity levels among African American and disadvantaged women underscore the importance of developing interventions to promote physical activity and exercise that address the specific cultural values, beliefs, and practices of these women. The purpose of the present study was to identify cultural, environmental and policy determinants of physical activity to inform the development of exercise interventions for preventing CVD in low-income, urban African American women aged 20 to 50 years.

METHODS

Six focus groups were held, three at each of two federally funded community health centers serving a total of four communities on Chicago's West Side. The communities are predominantly African American (67.0% to 99.2%) and low income (median family income $9,336 to $24,877), and more than half the households are headed by women (50.4% to 74.5%) (CDPH, 2000). All list heart disease as the major cause of death. The communities rank 3rd, 5th, 7th, and 16th of 77 Chicago communities on heart disease mortality (City of Chicago, 1994).

The study received approval from the institutional review board at the University of Illinois at Chicago. Potential participants were informed of the study by flyers posted at the health centers and a local daycare center. Women were also informed through health care staff, a community outreach worker from one of the health centers and word-of-mouth. All recruiters were trained by the research staff in recruitment procedures. Interested women either called the research offices or agreed to give their name, address, and telephone number to the contact person for a telephone call from the staff. During the telephone call a staff member further explained the study and screened each woman for eligibility. In addition to age (20 to 50 years) and physical inactivity (no regular leisure time physical activity), women had to identify themselves as African American. Women were encouraged to inform their friends of the study. A reminder telephone call was made to the women the day before their scheduled participation. Those who arrived at the focus group but had not been screened earlier were informed of the study and screened on site. Three focus groups included women aged 20 to 35 years; the other three, women 36 to 50 years.

Before the focus group actually began, each woman was again informed individually about the study, and a member of the research staff read the consent form to her. An experienced female African American nurse researcher/clinical psychologist moderated all six focus groups. A nurse practitioner/researcher served as assistant moderator and operated the tape recorder, handled environmental conditions and logistics, and took notes. Lunch or breakfast was provided. After the discussion the moderator read demographic questions to participants, who filled in their responses; each woman received $20 at the completion of the session. Assistance was provided to women who could not read. The moderator and assistant moderator debriefed each other at the completion of each focus group.

The sessions were tape-recorded and transcribed in their entirety by an experienced transcriber and transcripts were read and coded by three researchers independently. After the results were compared and a consensus reached, the transcripts and codes were entered into QSR NUD*IST qualitative software. The research team met to discuss impressions and reach consensus on themes related to the concepts of culture, environment, and policy.

Forty-eight women participated in the six focus groups (range 5 to 11). Most participants (85%) were unmarried, 40% had less than a high school education, and 33% were neither employed nor attending school. On average, 5.27 persons were living in their household (range, 1-19; SD, 3.59) with a mean of 2.89 children under 18 living there (range, 0-15; SD, 2.94). No significant differences between sites were found by marital status, education, employment, or number of children.

RESULTS

Culture

Across all age groups the participants described three types of women: the physically active, the physically inactive, and the exerciser. The physically active woman's entire day was filled with activities. Involved with her world and the lives of others, particularly her children and grandchildren, she rose early and spent her day taking children to and from school, doing laundry, "constantly fixing something to eat," "chasing kids all day," making sure they were up for school, playing with them, and overseeing their safety and care. Time was spent running up and down stairs at home and at work. The physically active woman was involved in social groups, and religion was an integral part of her life. As one woman commented:

> She's spending her time in praise and worship. God and praise takes a lot of strength, you know. Hallelujah all over the place. That's what I would see that would take her through her day.

The physically active woman was "always on the go" and "meeting goals for a lot of people." Her hallmark was being engaged.

In contrast, the inactive woman had difficulty getting out of bed in the morning and was not engaged with the world. Although she had children, they also "slept late." This was the woman who "wakes up just in time for the soap operas" and then may return to bed. If she goes outside she "just sits there . . . stuck." The inactive women "do nothing all day." Unlike the active woman, she was someone with "low self-esteem" and limited "energy" and was unemployed.

The exerciser was described as an organized woman who engaged in leisure time activity such as jogging, biking, or aerobics or who used exercise equipment regularly. The exerciser was portrayed as consuming very small quantities of food or eating only healthy food.

> Probably drinking some coffee in the morning . . . a piece of toast and do exercise. She probably would eat carrots and celery, lettuce . . . you know, stuff like that for lunch. She would eat a small amount because her stomach is probably already that size.

The focus group participants described the African American women they knew as being either "physically active" or "physically inactive," not "exercisers." Most believed that they were personally among the physically active. They suggested, however, that lack of community support and scarcity of role models were cultural influences that discouraged them and other African American women from being exercisers. They were not encouraged by women in their own socioeconomic group to engage in exercise, and they did not see women in their neighborhood walking or jogging. They feared being teased if they exercised in public because they were not physically fit; the teasing would be devastating to their self-esteem.

Some women found it easy to compare and contrast the physical activity of women from different cultures, but others saw it as stereotyping. Some believed they had little information about different cultures and thus did not feel competent to state an opinion. As expected, they were knowledgeable about women from the dominant culture (Caucasian), with whom they had the most contact, as well as women of Mexican descent. They had little familiarity with Asian and American Indian women. Their description of the exerciser was consistent with their view of Caucasian women, whom they saw as "jogging all the time," "really getting into it . . . skating and everything" and "riding them bikes." They suggested the dominant culture could financially afford to free themselves from chores, such as cooking and cleaning, and thus have time for exercise. Although Mexican women were not seen as exercisers, they were perceived as having the benefit of female group cohesiveness. They "stuck together" and supported one another in taking on a variety of behaviors that could extend to exercise. Asian women were also not seen as exercisers, but as a group they were seen as "thin" because of their eating habits and a genetic predisposition. As a woman commented, "You don't see a lot of fat Asians and that might be because they don't believe in eating a lot of things."

Safety was an issue. They expressed the opinion that African American women were not provided the same protection to exercise freely in their communities as women from the dominant culture. For example:

They (Caucasian women) have more protection in their neighborhoods than we do. I mean, they see somebody, you know, looking crazy and all of a sudden you got 20 cops coming out of somewhere. But we got about 50 people looking crazy in our neighborhood and don't nobody do nothing.

Environment

The environment of these women can be characterized by its extreme poverty and saturation with drugs and crime. Every group made reference to "drug dealers," "gangbangers," and bullets. Many women were reluctant to venture far from their own front porch, and some feared for the safety of their families even within their homes. One woman commented, "You know, they're fighting all the time and you might be the one to walk out the door and get hit or shot." On the other hand, some women mentioned refusing to be a "prisoner" in their homes, making attempts to say hello to everybody including "gangbangers," and pointing out that although people are selling drugs they "don't harass you."

Although they lived in the nation's third-largest city, with abundant opportunities for exercising along a lakefront with walking and running trails, they perceived these areas to be beyond their community boundaries. Most of their communities had parks, but although some felt safe in these parks many did not. One woman commented, "I have a park right across from my house, and I wouldn't go over there if you paid me." Another women felt comfortable taking her children to the park near her home. The women generally believed that facilities providing indoor activities were not easily accessible within their communities.

... either it's (the facility) in the middle of some place where you have to go through 12 gangs, 6 drug dealers just to get to 'em ... all before you get to the door. What's the point of even going?

Participants thought that the dominant culture was not providing adequate policing or sufficient protection of women and families in their community.

Public transportation, the major means of getting someplace within the community, was both an enabler of physical activity and a barrier to becoming more active. There was general consensus that transportation was readily accessible, and some women suggested that public transportation gave them an opportunity to become more active by running or walking fast for a block or two to catch the bus or train. Because few women had cars, they had to walk; as a grandmother said, "It's like I enjoy it (walking), you know. It's dragging the kids, but they getting used to it . . ." Other women, however, thought that ready access to public transportation discouraged them from walking to do their errands or go to work.

The women's homes also provided both enablers and barriers. The women frequently mentioned the availability and advantages of stairs within their homes and buildings for obtaining physical activity. Stairwells raised safety issues for some women who saw them as an area for drug dealers or addicts to congregate. Other hindrances to home exercise included having large numbers of people living there which limited both space and privacy.

Opportunities to be physically active in the work environment varied by job. Women with clerical positions said they "sat most of the day" and were often restricted in their movements. For example, a data processor commented, "You wait for somebody to come and let you go to the washroom and stuff." Other women performed physically demanding jobs, such as loading trucks for United Parcel Service. Many women had service jobs related to child and home care, which they suggested contributed to their being physically active. In general, they saw themselves as stronger than women from other ethnic groups, some suggesting that their ancestors' long history of slavery and "hauling bales of cotton" was the basis for their physical strength. The socio-cultural and physical environment and policy factors identified by these urban, low-income women that relate to physical activity are summarized in Table 1.

Interventions

The women were very vocal and creative in their view of the ideal physical activity intervention. Some suggested physical interventions and others socio-

TABLE 1. Factors Identified by Urban, Low-Income African American Women That Relate to Physical Activity

Socio-Cultural Environment	Physical Environment & Policy
Social Factors • mentioned the need for community support • had no role models • viewed physical activity as a group effort Cultural Factors • differentiated between physically active, inactive and exercising women • exercising was seen as a part of a Caucasian woman's culture • cited Caucasian women lived in safer neighborhoods and could exercise outdoors because of this	Physical Environment • no immediate access to places • places are beyond community boundaries Safety • lack of personal safety (e.g., from drug-dealers, gang members) Policy • work environments vary in level of physical activity • public transportation • cost issues

cultural interventions but they saw the two as necessary and complementary. Women from all the groups envisioned the development of a facility to meet their recreational needs, a facility that might have a sauna, a swimming pool, a sitting room with a TV, child care facilities, and a bar with juices and healthy snacks. Several groups were enthusiastic about beautifying an existing facility by cleaning, painting, wallpapering, or by creating a mural.

Of equal importance to developing convenient and appealing facilities was the women's desire for social support in their efforts to become more physically active. Interestingly, they viewed becoming physically active as a group effort and advocated that women work together to establish an "emotional connection" to increase "motivation." The theme was leading by example, as this comment suggests:

> ... somebody start walking ... see you walking and they may start walking ... you pick up people as you do that ... then it will build up.

They wanted to reach out to other women who were "overwhelmed with their everyday life" and "disconnected from the community and other women." They suggested using certificates and prizes to reward women and increase their sense of accomplishment and motivation. In addition to exercise opportunities, their ideal facility would provide counseling and classes in self-esteem, time management, job training, parenting, nutrition, gardening, cooking, and sewing. Additional comprehensive services would be provided for the entire family that were tailored to their needs.

Policy

For these women, policy development centered around safety issues, cost, availability, and community input. They wanted increased security in their neighborhoods so they could exercise publicly and go to exercise facilities without fear of harm. They desired an increased police presence, particularly in parks, to prevent them from being assaulted verbally or physically battered. In terms of cost, they knew that a facility offering exercise programs would require some sort of payment. They were willing to pay a fee but wanted affordable rates. They preferred a sliding scale on a monthly or pay-as-you-go basis and affordable or free child care to allow them time to exercise. They wanted facilities with extended hours to allow them to attend evenings and weekends, and they wanted facilities to be in their neighborhoods. One group discussed placing a facility in one of the vacant and abandoned lots scattered throughout its neighborhoods. Finally, they wanted policies in place to ensure that community members had input into the development and implementation of physical activity programs. The community needed to know that the program was for its own "benefit" and not just to "escalate the prestige" of the developer.

The women's socio-cultural, physical and policy intervention suggestions for physical activity are summarized in Table 2.

DISCUSSION

The Chicago focus groups were conducted with African American women who were primarily of low income and limited education, mostly unpartnered with many unemployed or working in a minimum-wage service position. Their daily lives were conducted within the context of their neighborhood, and they seemed to be outsiders in their view of the larger community of Chicago. Most considered themselves physically active and knew others in their neighborhood like themselves, but they did not personally know any women who exercised. Exercise was part of the culture of the Caucasian women they saw in those areas of the city that were beyond their borders. As in earlier findings, however, they understood the additional value of exercise in their daily lives and desired this for themselves (Nies, Vollman, & Cook, 1999; Eyler et al., 1998). Unfortunately, they did not readily identify resources for physical activity available to them in their communities.

Safety issues, limited finances, and lack of social support were identified as major barriers to exercise and becoming more physically active. These barriers are consistent with literature on the correlates of physical activity in women (King et al., 2000; Carter-Nolan, Adams-Campbell, & Williams, 1996; Johnson, Corrigan, Dubbert, & Gramling, 1990), but there was some difference for these low-income women. First, their concerns for safety were at the individual level, not at the physical environment level (e.g., lighting or sidewalks) with fears of being attacked or falling prey to a random bullet from a gun. Also, the homeless and mentally ill, whom the authorities apparently consider indig-

TABLE 2. Physical Activity Intervention Suggestions from Urban, Low-Income, African American Women

Socio-Cultural	Physical	Policy
• need role models to lead by example • reach out to physically inactive women • mentoring and support programs • community support • creative opportunities for activity	• facility for women only • need amenities included (juice bar, sauna, etc.) • surroundings need to be physically appealing • replace empty and vacant lots • needs to be within neighborhood	• need family facility with daycare and activities for all family members • improve safety • incentives • get community input • address cost barrier

enous to the community, presented the potential of verbal threats on the side-walks and in parks. There was a repeated plea for an increased presence from law enforcement. Although the women did not mention problems with adequate lighting, unsafe sidewalks, or busy traffic, all of which are reported as issues related to safety in previous studies (King et al., 2000), we speculate that these concerns may exist but are overshadowed by fears for immediate personal safety. As expected, lack of money presented a barrier to exercise, particularly in relation to the lack of appealing facilities and to fee schedules that were prohibitive.

Participants also lacked role models of women exercising within their communities. Furthermore, they anticipated criticism from other women and neighbors if they ventured outside for exercise. There was the sense they would feel out of place and reproached if they exercised, because it was not culturally accepted in their neighborhood. Unlike earlier studies suggesting the importance of social support from persons such as family members and friends (Johnson, Corrigan, Duber, & Gramling, 1990; Nies, Vollman, & Cook, 1999), these women desired community support for those persons who tried to become more active. They suggested coming together as women, much like a coalition, to provide this needed support. Furthermore, they desired a voice in the development of interventions at both the social and physical environmental level to ensure success in providing exercise opportunities for women like themselves. In addition, they expressed a desire for recreational facilities that were physically pleasant and provided amenities to which they were not accustomed.

Despite the socioeconomic disadvantages of the participants, they were very aware that increased security and pleasant and safe facilities and parks would not be enough to provide the impetus to become exercisers–they realized the need for a comprehensive approach to change behaviors. Interestingly, they expressed the need for increasing women's self-esteem through job training, parenting, nutrition and cooking classes. Moreover, at the heart of each focus group one could see the importance these women placed on the care and guidance of children and grandchildren. Only if all of these aspects of a woman's life were considered would she gain the motivation to take on new behaviors. Unlike prior studies that indicated disadvantaged women felt the need to compensate for physically demanding labor and home responsibilities with rest, our participants discussed the need for time management skills to incorporate exercise.

CONCLUSION

The use of focus groups illuminated the essence of these African American women's lives and gave voice to the barriers they saw to becoming more physically active as well as their desire for interventions tailored to their needs. Future work on interventions for low-income African American women needs to consider the significance of family and address the importance of increasing self-esteem. Additionally, the use of incentives such as certificates of accomplishment and pleasurable experiences such as massages, rarely available to low-income women, may provide a feeling of being connected with other women and improve their self-esteem. Policy issues related to safety and fee structures are basic essentials to consider in developing exercise interventions conjointly with low-income women whether African American or not.

REFERENCES

American Heart Association. (2000). High blood pressure statistics. Available at: *<http://www.americanheart.org/heart_and stroke_A_Z_guide/hbps.html>* Accessed February 12, 2001.

Barker, J. C., Morrow, J., Mitteness, L. S., Fuller-Thomson, E., Minkler, M., & Driver, D. (1998). Gender, informal social support networks, and elderly urban African Americans a profile of grandparents raising grandchildren in the United States. *Journal of Aging Studies, 12*, 199-222.

Behavioral Risk Factor Surveillance System. (1999). Neighborhood safety and the prevalence of physical inactivity–Selected States, 1996. *Morbidity and Mortality Weekly Report, 48*(07), 143-146.

Behavioral Risk Factor Surveillance System. (1995). Prevalence of recommended levels of physical activity among women–Behavioral Risk Factor Surveillance System, 1992. *Morbidity and Mortality Weekly Report, 44*(06), 105-107.

Cardinal, B. J., & Sachs, M. L. (1996). Effects of mail-mediated, stage-matched exercise behavior change strategies on female adults' leisure-time exercise behavior. *The Journal of Sports Medicine and Physical Fitness, 36*, 100-107.

Carter-Nolan, P. L., Adams-Campbell, L. L., & Williams, J. (1996). Recruitment strategies for black women at risk for noninsulin-dependent diabetes mellitus into exercise protocols: A qualitative assessment. *Journal of The National Medical Association, 88* (9), 558-562.

Chen, A. H., Sallis, J. F., Castro, C. M., Lee, R. E., Hickman, S. A., & Martin, J. E. (1998). A home-based behavioral intervention to promote walking in sedentary ethnic minority women: Project WALK. *Journal of Women's Health: Research on Gender, Behavior, and Policy, 4*(1), 19-39.

Eyler, A. A., Baker, E., Cromer, L., King, A. C., Brownson, R. C., & Donatelle, R. J. (1998). Physical activity and minority women: A qualitative study. *Health Education and Behavior, 25*(5), 640-652.

Johnson, C. A., Corrigan, S. A., Dubbert, P. M., & Gramling, S. E. (1990). Perceived barriers to exercise and weight control practices in community women. *Women and Health, 16*(3-4), 177-191.

Krummel, D. A., Koffman, D. M., Bronner, Y., Davis, J., Greenlund, K., Tessaro, I., Upson, D., & Wilbur, J. (2001). Cardiovascular health interventions in women:

What works? *Journal of Women's Health and Gender-Based Medicine, 10*(2), 117-136.

Lasco, R. A., Curry, R. H., Dickson, V. J., Powers, J., Menes, S., & Merritt, R. K. (1989). Participation rates, weight loss, and blood pressure changes among obese women in a nutrition-exercise program. *Public Health Reports, 104*(6), 640-646.

King, A. C., Castro, C., Wilcox, S., Eyler, A. A., Sallis, J. F., & Brownson, R. C. (2000). Personal and environmental factors associated with physical inactivity among different racial-ethnic groups of U. S. middle aged and older-aged women. *Health Psychology, 19*(4), 354-364.

National Heart Lung and Blood Institute, Expert panel on the identification, evaluation, and treatment of overweight and obesity in adults. (1998). *Clinical Guidelines on the Identification, Evaluation and Treatment of Overweight and Obesity in Adults: The Evidence Report*. Bethesda, MD: National Heart, Lung and Blood Institute.

Nies, M. A., Vollman, M., & Cook, T. (1999). African American women's experiences with physical activity in their daily lives. *Public Health Nursing, 16*(1), 23-31.

U.S. Department of Health and Human Services. (2000). *Healthy People 2010 Objectives Volume II*. Washington, DC: Office of Disease Prevention and Health Promotion. ISBN 0-16-050499-6.

Environmental, Policy, and Cultural Factors Related to Physical Activity in Well-Educated Urban African American Women

Deborah Rohm Young, PhD
Xiaoxing He, MPH
Jeanette Harris
Iris Mabry, MD, MPH

SUMMARY. The purpose of this qualitative study was to identify environmental, policy, and cultural predictors of physical activity in urban African American women living in Baltimore, MD. Thirty-nine mostly well-educated women participated in eight focus group discussions, five

Deborah Rohm Young is affiliated with the University of Maryland, Department of Kinesiology, College Park, MD. Xiaoxing He and Jeanette Harris are affiliated with the Welch Center for Prevention, Epidemiology, and Clinical Research, Johns Hopkins University. Iris Mabry is affiliated with the Department of Pediatrics, Johns Hopkins Medical Institutions.

Address correspondence to: Deborah Rohm Young, University of Maryland, Department of Kinesiology, 2312 Health and Human Performance Building, College Park, MD 20742 (E-mail: dryoung@wam.umd.edu).

The authors acknowledge the contributions of Ms. Nadiyah Mohammed and Ms. Bernice Carey, who moderated the focus groups, Ms. Donna Moore, Ms. Areh Osaji Howell, Mr. Tavon English, and Ms. Sarah Allen, who helped schedule and organize the focus groups, and Ms. Elaine Lewis, who transcribed the focus groups. The authors also thank the focus group participants, who generously gave their opinions.

This project was funded by CDC SIP5-99.

[Haworth co-indexing entry note]: "Environmental, Policy, and Cultural Factors Related to Physical Activity in Well-Educated Urban African American Women." Young, Deborah Rohm et al. Co-published simultaneously in *Women & Health* (The Haworth Medical Press, an imprint of The Haworth Press, Inc.) Vol. 36, No. 2, 2002, pp. 29-41; and: *Environmental, Policy, and Cultural Factors Related to Physical Activity in a Diverse Sample of Women: The Women's Cardiovascular Health Network Project* (ed: Amy A. Eyler) The Haworth Medical Press, an imprint of The Haworth Press, Inc., 2002, pp. 29-41. Single or multiple copies of this article are available for a fee from The Haworth Document Delivery Service [1-800-HAWORTH, 9:00 a.m. - 5:00 p.m. (EST). E-mail address: getinfo@haworthpressinc.com].

for women aged 36 to 50 years and three for women 20 to 35 years of age. Transcripts were analyzed using QSR NUD*IST qualitative software, and themes were identified. The discussions identified numerous opportunities and barriers for physical activity. The women reported being aware of physical activity resources and facilities available to them, but they lacked time and motivation to participate. Family responsibilities and duties unique to African American women were cited often. The results suggest that providing more environmental facilities may not be sufficient to increase physical activity in well-educated urban African American women. Intervention strategies that place value on family and cultural responsibilities should be considered. *[Article copies available for a fee from The Haworth Document Delivery Service: 1-800-HAWORTH. E-mail address: <getinfo@haworthpressinc.com> Website: <http://www.HaworthPress. com> © 2002 by The Haworth Press, Inc. All rights reserved.]*

KEYWORDS. Qualitative data, physical activity, African Americans, women

PURPOSE

African American women bear a heightened risk for cardiovascular disease (CVD), which continues to be the nation's leading cause of death. The prevalence of physical inactivity, an independent risk factor of CVD, is also high among African American women (Crespo, Keteyian, Heath, & Sempos, 1996). The purpose of this study was to identify socio-cultural, environmental, and policy factors that play an important role in determining physical activity behavior among urban, African American women. These factors can then be used to help design effective community-based interventions for increasing physical activity and thereby reducing cardiovascular risk.

METHODS

Focus group participants were recruited from predominately African American churches in Baltimore, MD, 64% of whose 650,000 residents are African American (U.S. Census Bureau, 2000). The most important social institution in the African American community, churches, preserve African American culture and traditions (Levin, 1984) and, thus, are an appropriate target for recruitment. Women aged 20-50 years were recruited from flyers placed in churches, by word of mouth, and from a list of women participating in a previous church-based physical activity trial. The one-page flyers described the focus groups and gave a contact telephone number to call for more information. The project staff screened interested women over the telephone to determine their eligibility. Those eligible and still interested were scheduled for a focus group session based on their age and availability. Participants were sent a post-card reminder and were called the day before as well as the day of the focus group, whenever possible. Participants were provided with refreshments and were paid $20 for their participation. If needed, transportation was provided.

Before beginning, participants completed a brief demographic and lifestyle questionnaire. The focus group meetings (two hours in length) were conducted at two churches, but participants were not necessarily members of those churches. Most focus groups were scheduled in the evening, although one was conducted on a Saturday morning. An African American woman trained in conducting focus group discussions moderated all the sessions. The moderator was familiarized with the moderator's guide and the purpose of the discussions. An African American notetaker also was present at each session to record nonverbal expressions and identify key themes. Informed consent and permission to audiorecord the sessions were obtained.

After audiotapes were transcribed, the transcripts were read and coded by trained research assistants who read them together and reached consensus on coding. The codes used were consistent with those employed by the other field centers (Eyler et al., 2002) in this project. Coding was verified by one of the investigators and entered into QSR NUD*IST qualitative software.

Thirty-nine of the 118 scheduled women (33%) participated in the focus group discussions. Last-minute scheduling conflicts was the primary reason for non-attendance. Five groups were conducted for women aged 36-50 years and three for women 20-35 years. Attendance ranged from two to nine participants. More than three-fourths of participants were employed full-time (76%) and 57% had attended at least some college; about one-third (38%) were married. The mean Body Mass Index calculated with self-reported height and weight was 29.5 and 88% reported their health as being good or better.

RESULTS

The eight focus groups had similar discussions regarding social, environmental, policy, and cultural factors related to physical activity among African American women. The younger and older focus group age groups discussed similar themes. Therefore, the results are presented for the groups as a whole rather than reporting separately by age group.

Social Environmental Issues

Role of the Family

The discussions included conversations on how family responsibilities influenced women's physical activity levels. The women identified family and household responsibilities as important opportunities for them to be active as well as important barriers. Daily household chores such as cleaning up, doing laundry, and taking care of the children were mentioned.

> I feel I get a lot of physical activity just cleaning up behind everybody else, up and down the stairs, and washing and cooking . . .

> I would like to exercise twice a day. If I could do that, I would be happy, but I get home so late. By the time I finish, . . . with my son . . .

Many of the women said that their priorities and personal physical activity patterns had changed dramatically once they became mothers. "That's the difference with my activity. I'm not sitting around doing nothing, but I'm not doing the things for me, just for me, it's for other people."

Although some women thought that those who lived alone and didn't have the responsibilities of children would be more active, some with this circumstance disagreed.

> Well, I guess it's easier for me to be lazier because of the fact that I don't have the children or the other people to clean up behind . . .

> Oh, I'm saying I'm just lazy when it comes to exercising, because I live alone, too, and I have the same opportunities she has. I just don't have maybe the desire or the willpower.

A few women without family responsibilities said they could exercise before work or in the evening and thought that those with families may have less time available.

The women perceived that family culture influenced preferences for physical activity. They indicated that in families with other priorities, the children are raised not to be physically active, and this follows to the next generation. Conversely, in families that devote time to physical activity, physical activity is more likely to continue as the children become adults.

Some women said the high prevalence of single mothers in the African American community was another barrier to physical activity.

Role of Others

When considering their current physical activity habits, the women stated that having a friend or group to exercise with had been motivating in the past and would be a motivator again.

I came back [from walking in the park] and I shared it with a girlfriend, and she said, 'Oh, ____, I want to go with you.' And so then we started going, being motivated had a lot to do with it.

Building a bond, a friendship, and having a support group was considered to be an important component of a physical activity program.

Having a friend to exercise with was also seen as a method of protection. "The last time I took a walk by myself, and the people and the comments that they were making when I was walking back, which discouraged me from going by myself. If you have a buddy, you can talk."

The women discussed the importance of appropriate role models to promote physical activity.

People do by what they see, and I would have to set the example. They would have to see me wear my tennis shoes to work and jogging, you know, or parking my car far down the parking lot and jogging up to the building or at least doing my speed, power walking, as they say.

Physical Environmental Issues

Opportunities

For the most part, these urban African American women perceived plenty of opportunities in their household, neighborhood or community, or their work site, to be physically active (see Table 1). Some of the women currently or previously exercised or walked during their lunch break. Some reported having exercise opportunities at their respective churches, living close to parks or lakes, and having safe neighborhoods in which to walk (although some others reported their neighborhoods were not safe).

It's like the opportunity is right there, and I just don't want it, don't take advantage of it.

Some women cited living in the city provided opportunities for physical activity. They perceived there were a variety of places to walk (e.g., at Baltimore's Inner Harbor, in the malls, on tracks, or at playgrounds) and that because the areas are busy and people are "out and about," it makes it easier. One woman stated, "(In a city), everybody's busy . . ., so I think being in a city because there's so many people, you feel a little more comfortable than a rural area." One woman without a car stated that because the city is so spread out, "It's easy for me to get physical activity by actually going to where I have to go."

TABLE 1. Factors Influencing Physical Activity Behavior Among Urban African American Women Living in Baltimore

Socio-Cultural Environment	Physical Environment & Policy
Social • would like someone to exercise with for motivation • also serves as protection • need appropriate role models Cultural • economic issues • cultural responsibilities • lack of prior experience • acceptance of larger body size • changing perceptions about physical activity	Physical • walking for transportation • weather, lack of daylight were barriers • know of many places readily available, just need to use them Policy • many places cost-prohibitive • need a better variety of places to go such as shopping malls, tennis courts • schedules prohibitive, need worksite programs

Most focus groups discussed types of readily available physical activity that do not cost money. Walking was mentioned as a free activity that can be performed anyplace. Other such examples were: walking the stairs at work and taking the long way to the ladies' room, using muscles while doing household chores, and taking advantage of the free facilities and programs available in the community (e.g., church exercise classes).

Environmental Barriers

Although many women reported living in safe neighborhoods or having safe places to exercise, safety was a concern. One woman commented on how easy it was to be active in her neighborhood because a park was a block away, although another participant reminded her "Yes, but you have to walk across a busy street to get there." Concern about crime was also mentioned. As one woman joked, "If I wanted to run, I gotta take my pit bull with me, you know, 'cause the yo's on the corner might, you know . . ." Generally, although there was concern about personal safety, most women could either readily identify safe places to be physically active or articulate a strategy to make the environment safer (e.g., walk with a dog, or in a group).

Although facilities were considered readily available, cost was sometimes a barrier. The women also stated that some facilities, like tennis courts, were not readily available where they lived. Cold weather and lack of daylight were also cited as barriers.

Policy Issues

Some of the discussions on what the women would do at their work site or in their neighborhood or community to increase physical activity had policy implications. Suggestions included the following: Have malls provide indoor walking, use resources at schools, have work sites provide exercise facilities and changing/shower facilities or discounts to athletic clubs, institute exercise-break lunch policies, provide bonuses to those who exercise, build recreation centers for kids and adults or revitalize those centers that have been closed down, and establish government grants for putting exercise equipment in the home (see Table 2).

Additional comments included scheduling and staffing concerns.

> I think if something was offered in the neighborhood seven days a week, then if you miss one night, you could always go the next night. A lot of times, aerobics is held two nights a week and that's it. Then you have to wait until the next week to go.

When exercise facilities were available, there was a sense it was important to have appropriate staffing.

> But there was never anybody there to train you or help you create an exercise program or weight program and that kind of made me lose my motivation for utilizing those facilities.

Cultural Issues

When asked about how differences in cultures might influence physical activity level, a common theme was that there were many similarities across cultures.

> For women, I think across the spectrum, they all do household chores and take care of the children and things like that, so that's probably very common, as an example of some type of activity . . .

> I don't think there's really a drastic difference. I think it's what the media puts out for us to view.

Financial Resources

The most common explanation for cultural differences in physical activity was economics. The women reported that the African American culture had less economic stability and less financial resources for leisure pursuits than other cultures. A younger woman said that people from other cultures who had more money have greater opportunities for physical activity, extending from having funds available for adults to join gyms to providing children with opportunities to play sports.

TABLE 2. Physical Activity Intervention Suggestions from Urban African American Women Living in Baltimore

Socio-Cultural	Physical	Policy
• Aerobic classes in churches • Organize walking groups • Offer programs everyday • Offer programs that involve family members • Provide competent, helpful instructors • Instructors come to house • Provide health lectures and motivational workshops • Support groups • Competitions with rewards • Inform community members of available resources • Recruit for programs using surveys	• Eliminate elevators and escalators • Build low-cost adult recreation centers • Open facilities that have been closed • Use vacant buildings for recreational activities	• Provide exercise program at work • Provide shower facilities • Provide lunch-time programs • Provide bonuses for exercising • Provide government assistance for home exercise equipment • Open malls for walking • Open schools for exercise programs

> And going to private schools, they have all of that. And it's sad that our public schools are cutting out physical education and art and stuff like that. I think that's wrong.

There were also discussions about differences in physical activity that may have more to do with differences in social class than culture.

> I think that when you get to high-income people, their cultures are alike. I think black people exercise, are just as physically active as white people who have the same economic level.

One woman also stated that there are different priorities across cultures for spending money. She stated, "If we want a pair of shoes, we may sacrifice something for that, but we won't do it for our health. We'll say, 'Oh, well, that can wait until next year, or next month.' Then, next month you're buying another pair of shoes."

Cultural Responsibilities

Participants stated that another primary reason African American women are not physically active is that they take on more responsibilities than other women. This was a theme that recurred numerous times in both age groups. As one woman in the group aged 35-50 stated:

We tend to bear more burdens when it comes to the family . . . I think it was just bred in us from years and years ago, and we just continue that from one generation to the other generation.

We, as African Americans, we were taught to put ourselves last. You care for the house, you care for the children, you care for others . . . We try to fit everything in, and you are the last, you suffer.

And I think that's the hardest thing with Black women, is to keep your balance, because once you get married and you have children, you kind of put yourself on the back burner, and that's the struggle.

Prior Experiences

Both the younger and older age groups of focus groups discussed how the prior circumstances of African American people influence overall preferences and decisions about physical activity. In response to perceived cultural differences, a younger women stated, "They [Caucasians] always, usually they raise their children in sports, so when you get older, you're used to playing soccer and everything else." A woman from the older focus groups relayed that experiences her parents had with racism influenced how much activity her family was involved in. She stated, "They did what they had to do to survive, so we just kinda picked up on that. Now if we had parents who were really active, we probably would continue it."

Body Size Preferences

A common perception in all the focus groups was that white women are active because they want to maintain slender bodies, both to look good and to keep their husbands. The acceptance of larger body sizes in the African American community was thoroughly discussed.

Perceptions About Current Physical Activity

Some discussions suggested that African American women are becoming more active.

In the year 2000, you find a lot of our black people are getting into more exercise now, because they want the good health, they want to look good.

Recommendations for Intervention

The women provided numerous environmental and policy level recommendations to increase the physical activity levels of African American women, summarized in Table 2. Most of the suggestions related to altering the social environment, such as providing group exercise programs in the community and organizing educational lectures to relay information on the importance of being physically active. An oft-mentioned recommendation for increasing physical activity in the African American community was to provide programs that appeal to families and children. This was viewed both as a way of including the family and as a method for supervising children.

> It's not always easy getting day care for toddlers or youngsters or pre-teens when you want to do extra activities like that. I would do something that would include the family and/or the children.

Exposure to role models was a common recommendation for promoting physical activity. Positive role models, personal appeals, motivational speakers, and workshops were considered potentially effective. When asked how they would encourage physical activity in their community if they were in positions of power, the women suggested they would need to be active themselves, let others in the community observe their activity (e.g., walking, wearing sneakers), and then encourage others to join them.

Fewer recommendations were made for changing the physical environment or changing policies to promote physical activity (see Table 2). Some of the women doubted that these suggestions would be enacted.

> That just seems unreal to me. What bosses . . . encourage their employees to take a 20-minute nap or relaxation time . . . that's unreal to me. Come on.

> Well, they're also installing a gym down at my building, but when are we going to have time to use it?

DISCUSSION

The Baltimore focus groups were conducted in groups of African American women who were, for the most part, well educated and employed. They articulated social, environmental, and policy-level opportunities and barriers that influenced their personal physical activity levels and those of other African American women. The women reported a variety of physical activity resources available to them in their home, at work, and in their neighborhoods and communities, but generally they were not taking advantage of them. These results suggest that providing more physical environmental structures may not be sufficient to increase the physical activity levels of African American women. A more in-depth exploration of cultural factors may provide greater insight as to which strategies would have maximal effectiveness.

Although the women identified some cultural, environmental, and policy barriers, they were not perceived to be major. Participants identified many available opportunities for physical activity that they simply did not take. For the most part, they told us the relevant barriers were being motivated to engage in physical activity and finding time given their family, work, and community responsibilities. These barriers have been reported in studies of women of all cultural backgrounds (King, Castro, Eyler, Wilcox, Sallis, & Brownson, 2000) and for persons who exercise regularly as well as those who are sedentary (King, Blair, Bild, Dishman, Dubbert, Marcus, Oldridge et al., 1992; Young & King, 1995).

Most of the cultural differences the women discussed were not ones easily addressed through targeted interventions. The difference in incomes between whites and African Americans, for example, is a major social issue extending far beyond physical activity, is of long duration, and continues to have negative consequences for the African American community. Although the African American women from our focus groups thought their burdensome responsibilities were unique to their culture, from the series of focus groups conducted as part of this study (Eyler & Vest, 2002; Evenson, Sarmiento, Macon, Tawney, & Ammerman, 2002; Richter, Wilcox, Greaney, Henderson, & Ainsworth, 2002; Thompson, Allen, Cunningham-Sabo, Yazzie, Curtis, & Savis, 2002; Wilbur et al., 2002) and from other studies (Young, Gittelsohn, Charleston, Felix-Aaron, & Appel, 2001), these clearly constitute a major barrier that extends to most women. Other cultural differences, such as perceptions of different body image, have been reported elsewhere, and they likely play a role in differences by race or ethnicity in physical activity levels (Kumanyika, Wilson, & Guilford-Davenport, 1993). The influence of the commonly perceived link between physical activity and slimness/weight control that may serve to subtly discourage physical activity in African American women who place a generally lower value on being slim needs to be explored. To truly understand potential cultural differences that influence the value placed on health behaviors, more in-depth studies are needed.

The women acknowledged that their family and household responsibilities, although often burdensome, do provide them with some physical activity. National policy makers recognize that moderate-intensity activity can be conducted in a variety of formats, including household chores, and can contribute to meeting the current physical activity recommendations (U.S. Department of Health and Human Services, 1996). We do not know how much activity the women were engaging in, however, or if it was of moderate intensity. It was clear from the discussions that the women recognized that they were not as physically active as they either would like to be or "should be." Intervention strategies should acknowledge that most women engage in physical activity as part of their daily routines but should encourage them to devote some time on a regular basis for themselves (i.e., in active recreational or leisure pursuits) as well.

One potentially fruitful intervention strategy to explore is to involve the family. Almost all of the focus groups had discussions that focused on how influential the family is both for providing opportunities and influencing future preferences for physical activity. Safe, low-cost family activities that provide for a variety of physical activity experiences for all ages can influence the next generation to enjoy physical activity as well as provide the current generation with physical activity opportunities.

CONCLUSION

In conclusion, the urban, well-educated, working African American women in this study identified opportunities for physical activity as well as barriers to being active. They reported ample resources and facilities for physical activity, but they lacked time and motivation to participate. Family responsibilities were viewed as both an opportunity and a barrier. Because of the high perceived value of fulfilling their family and community responsibilities, successful interventions will have to recognize the importance of this cultural value. Messages and strategies that reinforce how physical activity benefits the entire family and can provide women with additional personal resources (e.g., more energy, better health, improved time management) to better serve these responsibilities should be considered. From these focus groups, the discussions suggest that a conceptual model that includes personal, cultural, and environmental factors is appropriate to explain the physical activity of African American women.

REFERENCES

Airhihenbuwa, C. O., Kumanyika, S., Agurs, T. D., & Lowe, A. (1995). Perceptions and beliefs about exercise, rest, and health among African-Americans. *American Journal of Health Promotion*, *9*, (6), 426-429.

Evenson, K. R., Sarmiento, O. L., Macon, M. L., Tawney, K. W., & Ammerman, A. S. (2002). A qualitative study of physical activity determinants among Latina immigrants.

Eyler, A. A., Baker, E., Cromer, L., King, A. C., Brownson, R. C., & Donatelle, R. J. (1998). Physical activity and minority women: A qualitative study. *Health Education and Behavior*, *25*, (5), 640-652.

Eyler A. A., & Vest, J. R. (2002). Environmental and policy barriers to physical activity in rural white women. *Women & Health*, *36*, (2), 111-121.

Eyler, A., Wilcox, S., Matson-Koffman, D., Evenson, K., Sanderson, B., Thompson, J., Wilbur, J. E., & Young, D. R. (2002). Correlates of physical activity among women from diverse racial/ethnic groups: A review. *Journal of Women's Health and Gender-Based Medicine, 11,* (3), 239-253.

Flynn, K. J., & Fitzgibbon, M. (1998). Body images and obesity risk among black females: A review of the literature. *Annals of Behavioral Medicine, 20,* (1), 13-24.

King, A. C., Blair, S. N., Bild, D. E., Dishman, R. K., Dubbert, P. M., Marcus, B. H., Oldridge, N. B., Paffenbarger, R. S., Jr., Powell, K. E., & Yeager, K. K. (1992). Determinants of physical activity and interventions in adults. *Medicine and Science in Sports and Exercise, 24,* (6 Supplement), S221-S236.

Kumanyika, S., Wilson, J. F., & Guilford-Davenport, M. (1993). Weight-related attitudes and behaviors of black women. *Journal of the American Dietetic Association, 93,* (4), 416-422.

Levin, J. S. (1984). The role of the black church in community medicine. *Journal of the National Medical Association, 76,* (5), 477-483.

Morbidity and Mortality Weekly Reports. (1999). Neighborhood safety and the prevalence of physical inactivity–selected states, 1996. 48, (7), 143-146.

Richter, D. L., Wilcox, S., Greaney, M. L., Henderson, K. A., & Ainsworth, B. E. (2002). Environmental, policy, and cultural factors related to physical activity in African American women. *Women & Health, 36,* (2), 91-109.

Sallis, J. F., & Owen, N. (1998). Interventions to promote physical activity in communities and populations. In *Physical activity and behavioral medicine.* (pp.153-173), Thousand Oaks, CA: Sage Publications.

United States Census Bureau. (2000). <*http://www.census.gov.geo*>.

Thompson, J. L., Allen, P., Cunningham-Sabo, L., Yazzie, D. A., Curtis, M., & Davis, S. M. (2002). Environmental, policy, and cultural factros related to physical activity in sedentary American Indian women. *Women & Health, 36* (2), 59-74.

Young, D. R., Gittelsohn, J., Charleston, J., Felix-Aaron, K., & Appel, L. J. (2001). Motivations for exercise and weight loss among African American women: Focus group results and their contribution towards program development. *Ethnicity and Health, 6,* 227-245.

Young, D. R., & King, A. C. (1995). Exercise adherence: Determinants of physical activity and applications of health behavior change theories. *Medicine, Exercise, Nutrition, and Health, 4,* (4), 335-348.

Environmental, Policy, and Cultural Factors Related to Physical Activity Among Latina Immigrants

Kelly R. Evenson, PhD, MS
Olga L. Sarmiento, MD, MPH
M. Lisa Macon, BSPH
Kathy W. Tawney, PhD
Alice S. Ammerman, DrPH, RD

SUMMARY. According to national surveillance studies, participation in leisure-time physical activity remains low among minority women.

Kelly R. Evenson and Olga L. Sarmiento are affiliated with the Department of Epidemiology, School of Public Health, University of North Carolina-Chapel Hill, Chapel Hill, NC 27599-7435. M. Lisa Macon is affiliated with the Center for Health Promotion and Disease Prevention, University of North Carolina-Chapel Hill, Chapel Hill, NC 27599-7426. Kathy W. Tawney is affiliated with the Division of Nephrology and Hypertension, University of North Carolina Hospitals, Chapel Hill, NC 27599-7155. Alice S. Ammerman is affiliated with the Department of Nutrition, School of Public Health, University of North Carolina-Chapel Hill, Chapel Hill, NC 27599-7461.

Address correspondence to: Kelly R. Evenson, Department of Epidemiology, School of Public Health, University of North Carolina-Chapel Hill, 137 East Franklin Street, Suite 306, Chapel Hill, NC 27514 (E-mail: kelly_evenson@unc.edu).

The authors thank Erica Thompson, Jimmy Newkirk, and their corresponding staff and contacts for recruiting the participants and organizing the groups. The authors also thank Erika Campos, Melida Colindres, and Carmen Samuel-Hodge. The authors greatly appreciate the participation of the women in the focus groups.

This work was funded by the Centers for Disease Control and Prevention grant #U48/CCU409660 and by the Robert Wood Johnson Foundation grant #039361.

[Haworth co-indexing entry note]: "Environmental, Policy, and Cultural Factors Related to Physical Activity Among Latina Immigrants." Evenson, Kelly R. et al. Co-published simultaneously in *Women & Health* (The Haworth Medical Press, an imprint of The Haworth Press, Inc.) Vol. 36, No. 2, 2002, pp. 43-57; and: *Environmental, Policy, and Cultural Factors Related to Physical Activity in a Diverse Sample of Women: The Women's Cardiovascular Health Network Project* (ed: Amy A. Eyler) The Haworth Medical Press, an imprint of The Haworth Press, Inc., 2002, pp. 43-57. Single or multiple copies of this article are available for a fee from The Haworth Document Delivery Service [1-800-HAWORTH, 9:00 a.m. - 5:00 p.m. (EST). E-mail address: getinfo@haworthpressinc.com].

Furthermore, the correlates of such activity in this group are not well understood. To better understand the environmental, policy, and sociocultural correlates of physical activity among Latina immigrants, six focus groups were conducted in rural North Carolina. Among the 49 participants, median age was 32 years and median education 11 years. Participants were first generation immigrants from Mexico (n = 43), El Salvador (n = 3), Colombia (n = 1), the Dominican Republic (n = 1), and Honduras (n = 1). Environmental and policy barriers to activity were identified, including transportation, lack of facilities, cost, and safety. Sociocultural correlates of activity included gender roles for activity, importance of support from the family and husband, child care issues tied to having few relatives who lived close by, language, and isolation in the community. The women suggested changes and programs that could promote physical activity through multiple channels, especially involving the family. This information can be used to develop culturally appropriate interventions to increase physical activity among Latinas. *[Article copies available for a fee from The Haworth Document Delivery Service: 1-800-HAWORTH. E-mail address: <getinfo@haworthpressinc.com> Website: <http://www.HaworthPress.com> © 2002 by The Haworth Press, Inc. All rights reserved.]*

KEYWORDS. (MeSH terms): Emigration and immigration, exercise, focus groups, Hispanic Americans, leisure activities, women

PURPOSE

Information on the correlates of physical activity among Latinas (Latino women) is sparse, even though it is vital for the development of culturally appropriate physical activity interventions for this rapidly growing population. Estimates are that by 2010, Latinos will comprise the largest minority group in the U.S., and by 2050, one in four Americans will be Latino (Office of Minority Health and State Center for Health Statistics, 1999). In North Carolina, the Latino population growth rate has been double the rate for the total population (Johnson-Webb & Johnson, 1996). To better understand the environmental, policy, and sociocultural correlates of physical activity, we collected qualitative data among Latina first generation immigrants living in North Carolina, the 11th largest state by population in the U.S. according to the U.S. Census Bureau year 2000 data.

METHODS

The Office of Management and Budget (U.S. Census) defines Hispanic or Latino as a person of Cuban, Mexican, Puerto Rican, South or Central American, or other Spanish culture or origin regardless of race. For this study, the term Latina refers to women living in the U.S. whose origin is one of those listed. Focus group interviews with Latina immigrants were conducted during May and June 2000 in two North Carolina counties (one in the western and one in the eastern part of the state), chosen because of their prevalence of Latino immigrants. In the western county, women were recruited for focus groups through a local health center, an apartment complex, and a church. In the eastern county, women were recruited through several churches.

Of six focus groups in all, three were conducted among women 20 to 35 years old (two western and one eastern county) and three were conducted among women 36 to 50 years old (two eastern and one western county). Each focus group was comprised of 6 to 11 volunteer women who were not regular exercisers in the past 6 months (i.e., they did not exercise 3 or more times per week for at least 20 minutes each time). Each participant provided consent and received a fact sheet about the study, which was approved by the University of North Carolina-Chapel Hill School of Public Health and the CDC institutional review boards. At completion, participants received $20. Using a standardized focus group guide based on the socioecologic model (McLeroy, Bibeau, Stecker, & Glanz, 1988), the same experienced Latina moderator conducted all six focus groups. The guide contained questions on the correlates of physical activity and suggestions for interventions that addressed several levels of the socioecologic model (e.g., intrapersonal, interpersonal, community, and policy). All sessions were conducted in Spanish and a notetaker was always present. The conversations were audiotaped, and the contents were transcribed in Spanish, translated into English, then verified by a second native Spanish-speaking reviewer.

All qualitative data were independently double coded, with discrepancies between the two coders rectified. Data were analyzed using NUD*IST® (Nonnumerical, Unstructured, Data-Indexing, Searching, Theorizing). For each major theme analyzed, differences by location (eastern vs. western county) and age (20-35 vs. 36-50 years) were examined. Because differences by location and age were not identified, only pooled data are reported. Acculturation, defined as the transfer of culture from one group of people to another group of people (Negy & Woods, 1992), was assessed using a validated scale developed for Latinos (Marin, Sabogal, Marin, Otero-Sabogal, & Perez-Stable, 1987). This study was conducted in collaboration with the CDC Women's Cardiovascular Health Network. Additional details on the methodology are described elsewhere (Eyler et al., 2002).

RESULTS

Of the 49 participants, 25 lived in western and 24 lived in eastern North Carolina. Most were low-acculturated immigrants who were married with at least one child (see Table 3 in Eyler et al., 2002). Their median age was 32 years and median education 11 years. Most were from Mexico (n = 43), with three from El Salvador, and one each from Colombia, the Dominican Republic, and Honduras. The median level of acculturation was 1.9 (range, 1.0-3.4; SD, 0.65), with possible scores ranging from 1 (least acculturated) to 5 (most acculturated). Most women preferred to speak Spanish, which they often used with family and friends. Environmental, policy, and sociocultural correlates are summarized in Table 1 and are explored in depth below.

Environmental and Policy Correlates

Transportation: Many Latinas depended on their husband to drive them places, because they did not have a driver's license. A license was equated

TABLE 1. Sociocultural, Environmental, and Policy Factors Identified by Latinas that Relate to Physical Activity

Sociocultural	Environmental and Policy
Gender roles for activity • Sports are for men	Transportation • Not knowing how to drive • Lack of bus service
Importance of the family • Family comes before self • Lack of time for self because of household responsibilities	Lack of facilities • Lack of sidewalks • Parks not close to home • Schools closed for after-hours use
Husband support • Husband's value of physical activity	Cost • Fees for gym • Child care services
Child care • Relatives not close by to help	Safety • Afraid to walk alone • Unleashed dogs • Speeding traffic made walking on some roads dangerous • Felt unsafe in some outdoor parks
Language • Difficult to enroll in exercise classes if don't speak English	
Isolation in the community • Not notified of programs or opportunities in the community • Looked at strangely when out in the community	

with freedom, as it reduced reliance on spouses and others for help with transportation. Because physical activity facilities were often not located near the women's home, the transportation required was a barrier to being more active.

> Sometimes we are conformists. We just accept that we do not have time to do everything. In my case, in Mexico, when I was little I used to exercise–aerobics. Since I arrived here, it has been difficult because I don't drive and I can't go anywhere by myself.

> Yes, because there are women who can't leave their homes because they can't drive. If their husband does not take them to the store then they can't even go outside.

> . . . Here [in North Carolina], now things are a little bit different because there are more Hispanics, but in the past I used to feel very happy when I saw other Hispanics in the area. I think that I was the first Hispanic woman to drive in this area. Now you see more Hispanic women driving. But now, actually now, it is very nice to see more women driving because that means that they have more freedom. I used to be one of those women who had to wait for their husbands to get home to go out because I didn't know how to drive, until one day when I said to myself I have to learn how to drive for my own good–for my children and for my husband, too, because that way I can help them.

Local bus transportation was not available in either county, whereas it was available and frequently used by the women in their home country.

> Another thing is that I don't like to drive in my [home] country. I used to take the bus everywhere because it was easier than driving and finding a parking space. I think that if we had better transportation services here we would walk to the bus stop and we would use cars less.

Lack of Facilities: All of the focus group discussions included comments on lack of sidewalks and parks close to home. Few destinations or close places to walk and speeding traffic were deterrents to physical activity. Local schools had physical activity facilities, but these facilities could not always be utilized by the women.

> Another thing, here you can't go running around the track at the public schools. They won't give you permission, or the police will give you a ticket and will ask you to leave, or they will be closed.

Cost: Cost was a barrier for some women. The few gyms that were available were expensive to attend. Almost all groups mentioned cost as another barrier.

> I am 36 years old. Women of our age are raised physically and mentally in different ways. That's the reason why we don't take time for us. However, some women can set up a schedule and can afford to do exercise. You need money for everything. Some people have the money. Therefore, they can keep their body and mind physically active. Maybe it is the money.

Safety: The women mentioned a need to increase safety in some of the existing outdoor parks. Feeling insecure in this new country was commonly expressed.

> In Mexico it is different. Where I'm from, every afternoon kids go outside to play soccer, they eat on the streets, they really enjoy it. Here you can't go outside because a car can run over you or the kids can get robbed.

> Sometimes I tell my husband that I am going to walk to the church, because I don't have anybody to take me there. However, my husband says not to go because it is not the same like in our country [Mexico]. Here it is more dangerous [to walk in North Carolina] than in our country.

A fear of unleashed dogs was a safety barrier to walking outside in some neighborhoods.

> . . . Last time I was walking and a dog almost bit me. They have their dogs in the yard without a leash. I think they should tie up their dogs.

Sociocultural Correlates

Gender Roles for Activity: Participation in structured exercise was not always a part of the Latinas' cultural upbringing in her native country. In general, Latino boys were encouraged to play sports, such as soccer, while the girls were not encouraged to play sports. In fact, some women recalled that as girls they were discouraged from engaging in physical activities other than those related to housework and family responsibilities.

> And also, it is not part of our culture, physical exercises are for men, there are just a few athletic women.

Importance of the Family: The theme of the family was pervasive in all focus groups. The children, husband, and household duties came before the woman's personal needs. Similarly, the family's health came before her own.

I think that for Latino women the family is very important and I think that it is more important for us to take care of the kids than to exercise. The family is more important than exercise.

For example, my mother always kept us active. We were cleaning and ironing. We were always active at home. My mom never told us, "Wait an hour for me because I have to go to the gym."

Lack of time was often cited as a barrier to physical activity, because taking care of their families and household responsibilities were a higher priority. Several women who worked stated that when they arrived home they were expected to cook and take care of the children, which left little time for themselves.

I only walk, but when the baby sleeps I do my house duties. When the baby is awake, I prefer to play with him and I don't have time for anything else.

We have too much work at home; we need to find some time for ourselves.

Our husbands are relaxing and we are doing the household work. We continue working after working [referring to household work after coming home from their jobs].

Husband Support: Some women had husbands who were supportive of their physical activity, but most did not. Some of the men did not value physical activity for their wives and they described their husbands as desiring to see the house clean and having dinner ready when they arrived home from work.

The Latino men always say, "Women at home and men at work. You don't need to exercise."

Sometimes he [my husband] has to do something or he doesn't like to arrive home when I am not there. He wants everything clean and the food ready. Well, you know, they're working the whole day. They are tired and they like to see everything clean in the house.

Child Care: Child care was a challenge for some women, especially because many left their extended family in the home country. Some women did not trust persons outside their extended family to care for their children.

Yes, I agree, because most of us only have our husband and kids here. However, there are others who are more fortunate and have their mother

> or mother-in-laws to help them with the kids. Most of us are by ourselves and it is difficult to find someone to take care of the kids.

> We don't trust anybody to take care of our children.

> In this state we don't have a sport center for Hispanic women, a place where we can go for free, that is what we would like because we can't leave our children without food just to pay for a place where we can exercise to become pretty.

Language: All groups discussed being unable to speak English as a barrier to participating in community physical activity programs.

> Because they [Americans] were born here, they can speak the language. Therefore, they are able to register in any place easily. It is more difficult for us, because we don't know what to say.

> For example, the gyms here, one of the barriers is the language. If you register and they don't have an instructor that speaks Spanish . . . although there are some very brave women who register without speaking English. I talked to a friend who used to go when she was single.

Isolation in the Community: Some women mentioned feeling like outsiders which kept them from being more involved in activities outside their home.

> I have realized that people look at us strangely. Yes, here people are not used to seeing people from another country. They hear us talking and they start to look at us strangely. We feel bad, because they look at us strangely. Why are you looking at us that way? We are not bugs.

> We also feel isolated, to some extent, because not all of us tend to be free to do what we want. A lot of us feel isolated and dominated.

Interventions Recommended by Participants

The following channels were mentioned at least once as avenues for delivery of a physical activity intervention: churches, health departments, laundry rooms, schools, hospitals, work sites, and neighborhoods. Information learned in these environments could be disseminated through friends to reach the women at home and can involve the family.

> We probably won't read the information. We usually get the information through our friends . . . However, when we get the information through

other sources we really ignore it. We feel like it is not for us. We don't feel like we are included in any public information.

I think we have to reach the Latino community, just like what you did with this meeting. You went to find the people.

Environmental, policy, and sociocultural interventions suggested by the women in the focus groups are described below and summarized in Table 2.
Environmental and Policy Interventions: Public transportation was viewed as a way to give women more access to community activity opportunities.

TABLE 2. Sociocultural, Environmental, and Policy Intervention for Increasing Physical Activity Among Latinas

Sociocultural	Environmental & Policy
Knowledge of physical activity • Conduct information sessions or "charlas"	Transportation • Provide public transportation
Education • Improve education level of Latinas • Target educational programs specifically to men	Unleashed Dogs • Develop or enforce leash laws Lack of facilities • Provide more sidewalks • Provide more parks • Open outdoor school facilities to the public
Gym • Provide bilingual instructors and instructions • Offer programs tailored and targeted for Latinas	Worksite • Provide work time to be active • Subsidize health club fees • Provide incentives to be active
Family • Provide activities for the family to do together	
Neighborhood and Community • Promote walking groups • Reciprocal child care • Field trips to places in community to be active	
Social support • Increase support of husband by engaging a peer or mentor • Increase social networks among women	

And here [North Carolina], either you don't have a car or you do not have a driver's license. Therefore, you can't go wherever you want. I would like to have more public transportation services available.

All of the groups suggested having more facilities and local physical activity opportunities, including sidewalks and parks. Local schools could allow the use of indoor and outdoor facilities, thus promoting activity with existing community resources. Activities that could be undertaken as a family were mentioned often as a crucial component of any intervention.

I would think about providing a place with many rooms and also a pool. It is a good way for families to exercise together.

For example, I would have a park where people can bring their kids to play and run.

Policy interventions were mentioned less often, and most were related to the work site. Some women suggested providing work time to be active, such as during lunch breaks. Others mentioned that workplaces could subsidize health club fees or provide bonuses or incentives to be active.

When I worked in the health department they had a policy. If during your break you chose to go for a walk, they gave us 20 minutes, otherwise we had 15 minutes. Many of us chose to have only 15 minutes [women laughing]. Sometimes they gave us two breaks and we use them to go for a walk instead of sitting and drinking cola.

Sociocultural Interventions: Information on benefits of physical activity was requested through meetings or "charlas." Participants indicated that brief and clear messages were key. They also mentioned that formal education, such as completing their high school degree, would help women.

[Regarding an intervention] I think education is important, because when a woman is educated she will motivate herself for everything, because she can value herself.

The women suggested providing information in simple and clear Spanish, or in both Spanish and English. Bilingual instructors in gyms and bilingual instructions on equipment would also be helpful.

Participants emphasized that interventions to increase physical activity should include the family, not just the woman herself. Some women said they would appreciate child care, but it would have to be with someone they trusted.

Others mentioned they would rather engage in activities with their children than leave the caretaking to someone else.

> I think it will work when you get the whole family to participate in any activity.

> While we are exercising, we need to have activities for the kids, too. That will create a discipline for them and for us.

Women valued positive support from their husbands and consent from them to be more physically active. For this to happen, they suggested education directed to their husbands, which would be more effective from a male role model, perhaps a lay health advisor, than through wives or women in general.

> I think the information should be given to both men and women. That way they [men] will understand the benefits of being healthy.

> Involve them [husbands] in the system or have an active plan for the whole family.

Most groups stressed the leadership needed to help organize and motivate one another. Setting up a system of social support involving their social networks is an important piece to any intervention approach in their view.

> . . . The problem is that we don't know how to organize ourselves.

> We need to organize a group in such a way that some of us can take care of the kids while we exercise. We should help each other.

DISCUSSION

This qualitative study of Latina immigrants revealed many environmental, policy, and sociocultural enablers and barriers to physical activity. The themes identified were similar across two geographically distinct counties in North Carolina and across age (20 to 35 and 36 to 50 years). Many interventions to increase physical activity were suggested, with an emphasis on the importance of family involvement for a successful intervention.

The correlates of activity the women reported paralleled many factors described in other focus groups of women. Environmental barriers to activity have included safety and poor access (e.g., cost, lack of transportation and programs) (Eyler et al., 1998). The sociocultural correlates that make this study unique were related to the participants' being first-generation Latina immigrants with mainly low acculturation, a process involving changes in a person's values, beliefs, attitudes, and behaviors (Negy & Woods, 1992; Portes & Zhou, 1993). Challenges facing an immigrant woman include loneliness, social isolation, dependency on her husband or others for transportation, and lack of nearby relatives (Viadro, 1997). Any intervention that encourages social support from family and friends appears to be welcome in this population and might help ameliorate stress at the same time. During the process of acculturation, women may be weighing decisions to become more physically active, and this critical period of transition may be an opportune time for planning interventions to develop healthy and lasting new habits (King, 1994). The process of adaptation to a new culture can be very stressful.

Several other sociocultural barriers to physical activity were reported among our focus groups; the literature shows that these barriers affect other health behaviors as well. Not speaking English was often mentioned; some women who did not speak English lacked the confidence to attend activity classes or enroll at a gym. Conversely, participants perceived that speaking English gave them more freedom to make decisions and choices in their new country, thereby empowering them. Not surprisingly, other studies of Latinos have found that speaking English was a barrier to receiving health care services (National Coalition of Hispanic Health and Human Services Organizations, 1995; Scharer, 1999). Another barrier was lack of transportation and the women being dependent on husbands to take them places. This barrier has also been identified as a barrier to health care for Latinos (Scharer, 1999). Finally, the importance of the family was pervasive in our analysis, as has been noted elsewhere (National Coalition of Hispanic Health and Human Services Organizations, 1995). Effective, culturally competent interventions should involve the family. Intervention messages should emphasize the benefits to the family rather than the individual woman.

Only a few physical activity intervention studies in the literature have targeted Latinas (Avila & Hovell, 1994; Chen et al., 1998; Grassi, Gonzalez, Tello, & He, 1999; Nader et al., 1989) and thus formative data from the present study should be especially important in developing effective interventions. Regardless, any intervention should maximize the positive effects and minimize the negative aspects of acculturation. In reviewing the barriers to physical activity, we found that many were modifiable and could be addressed through interventions the women suggested.

Suggestions from participants also highlight the importance of developing interventions that fit easily into a daily routine. Small groups of women could be introduced to meet regularly, to be active with their families, and to be provided with support and information about other community services. For many women, their physical surroundings were new, and they mentioned not feeling confident in exploring new places. One possible strategy to promote physical activity is hosting field trips, which could include introducing the women to new places to be active (e.g., parks, walking trails at schools, gyms) while providing an initial experience with a supportive group. These interventions might increase their physical activity and also foster connections in their community. Fostering neighborhood walking groups and the use of reciprocal child care could also allow more women time to be active and also foster relationships with friends and family.

At the conclusion of the focus groups, many women asked for more information on physical activity, diet, and other risk factors for cardiovascular disease. Clearly, there was an unmet need for health information. Because physical activity behaviors are intertwined with other healthy behaviors, interventions should address other health issues and acculturation concerns as well. A physical activity intervention could help ease the transition process by relieving stress and bringing women together in a supportive environment.

Limitations

Qualitative data such as these can add substantially to our understanding of the correlates of physical activity among Latinas. Several limitations of this work should be acknowledged, however. The generalizability of the focus groups may be limited, as the women were volunteers from just two of North Carolina's 100 counties and were mainly women of modest education who were mostly from Mexico. Nationally, as well as in North Carolina, Hispanics of Mexican descent make up the largest Latino group (Office of Minority Health and State Center for Health Statistics, 1999). It is not known whether responses would have differed if the participants were mainly from other Latin American countries or if they had more education. There may be other physical activity correlates not addressed in these particular focus groups, especially among women who are regularly active or among Latinas who were born in the U.S. Even so, this study addresses a gap in the literature that can lead to more effective and appropriate interventions for Latinas. Finally, we should note that meaning or context may sometimes be lost when translating the women's quotes from Spanish to English.

CONCLUSION

This analysis indicates that many environmental, policy, and sociocultural correlates to physical activity and corresponding interventions to address these were identified with consistency across geographic location and age group.

This information will be used to develop a quantitative survey to further understand the correlates of physical activity among a larger group of Latinas. This work, in turn, will provide a framework for developing interventions to increase physical activity among Latinas.

REFERENCES

Avila, P., & Hovell, M. (1994). Physical activity training for weight loss in Latinas: A controlled trial. *Intl J Obes Relate Metabolic Disorders, 18*(7), 476-482.

Chen, A., Sallis, J., Castro, C., Lee, R., Hickmann, S., Williams, C., & Martin, J. (1998). A home-based behavioral intervention to promote walking in sedentary ethnic minority women: Project WALK. *Women Health, 4,* 19-39.

Eyler, A., Baker, E., Cromer, L., King, A., Brownson, R., & Donatelle, R. (1998). Physical activity and minority women: A qualitative study. *Health Ed Behavior, 25,* 640-652.

Eyler, A., Matson-Koffman, D., Vest, J., Evenson, K., Sanderson, B., Thompson, J., Wilbur, J., Wilcox, S., & Rohm Young, D. (2002). Environmental, policy, and cultural factors related to physical activity in a diverse sample of women: The Women's Cardiovascular Health Network Project–introduction and methodology. *Women & Health, 36*(2), 1-15.

Grassi, K., Gonzalez, M., Tello, P., & He, G. (1999). La vida caminando: A community-based physical activity program designed by and for rural Latino families. *J Health Ed, 30*(2), S-13-S-17.

Johnson-Webb, K., & Johnson, J. (1996). North Carolina communities in transition: An overview of Hispanic in-migration. *NC Geographer, 5,* 21-40.

King, A. (1994). Clinical and community interventions to promote and support physical activity participation. In R. Dishman (Ed.), *Advances in Exercise Adherence* (pp. 183-212). Champaign, IL: Human Kinetics.

Marin, G., Sabogal, F., Marin, B., Otero-Sabogal, R., & Perez-Stable, E. (1987). Development of a short acculturation scale for Hispanics. *Hisp J Behav Sci, 9*(2), 183-205.

McLeroy, K., Bibeau, D., Stecker, A., & Glanz, K. (1988). An ecologic perspective on health promotion programs. *Health Ed Q, 15*(4), 351-377.

Nader, O., Sallis, J., Patterson, T., Abramson, I., Rupp, J., Senn, K., Atkins, C., Roppe, B., Morris, J., Wallace, J., & Vega, W. (1989). A family approach to cardiovascular risk reduction: Results from the San Diego Family Health Project. *Health Ed Q, 16*(2), 229-244.

National Coalition of Hispanic Health and Human Services Organizations. (1995). Meeting the health promotion needs of Hispanic communities. *Am J Health Promot, 9*(4), 300-311.

Negy, C., & Woods, D. (1992). The importance of acculturation in understanding research with Hispanic-Americans. *Hisp J Behav Sci, 14*(2), 224-247.

Office of Minority Health and State Center for Health Statistics. (1999). *North Carolina Minority Health Facts: Hispanics/Latinos.* Raleigh, NC.

Portes, A., & Zhou, M. (1993). The new second generation: Segmented assimilation and its variants. *Ann Am Acad Political Soc Sci, 530,* 74-96.

Scharer, J. (1999). *Hispanic/Latino Health in North Carolina: Failure to Communicate?* Raleigh, North Carolina: NC Center for Public Policy Research.

Viadro, C. (1997). *Sexually transmitted diseases and married Hispanic immigrants in North Carolina: An exploration of social context, within-group differences, and methodology.* Dissertation, UNC-Chapel Hill, Chapel Hill, North Carolina.

Environmental, Policy, and Cultural Factors Related to Physical Activity in Sedentary American Indian Women

Janice L. Thompson, PhD
Peg Allen, MPH
Leslie Cunningham-Sabo, PhD, RD
Dedra A. Yazzie
Michelle Curtis, BA
Sally M. Davis, PhD

SUMMARY. Focus group interviews were conducted to explore sociocultural, environmental, and policy-related determinants of physical activity among sedentary American Indian women. Thirty women aged 20 to 50 years (mean = 37.4 ± 10.6 years) participated. Three sessions were

Janice L. Thompson is affiliated with The Office of Native American Diabetes Programs, University of New Mexico Health Sciences Center, Albuquerque, NM 87110. Peg Allen is affiliated with the Cancer Research and Treatment Center, Epidemiology and Cancer Control, University of New Mexico Health Sciences Center, Albuquerque, NM 87131. Leslie Cunningham-Sabo, Dedra A. Yazzie, Michelle Curtis and Sally M. Davis are affiliated with the Center for Health Promotion and Disease Prevention, The University of New Mexico Health Sciences Center, Albuquerque, NM 87131.

Address correspondence to: Janice L. Thompson, PhD, The Office of Native American Diabetes Programs, University of New Mexico Health Sciences Center, 1720 Louisiana Boulevard, Suite 312, Albuquerque, NM 87110 (E-mail: jthompson@salud.unm. edu).

Funding: U48/CCU 610818-05 from the Centers for Disease Control and Prevention.

[Haworth co-indexing entry note]: "Environmental, Policy, and Cultural Factors Related to Physical Activity in Sedentary American Indian Women." Thompson, Janice L. et al. Co-published simultaneously in *Women & Health* (The Haworth Medical Press, an imprint of The Haworth Press, Inc.) Vol. 36, No. 2, 2002, pp. 59-74; and: *Environmental, Policy, and Cultural Factors Related to Physical Activity in a Diverse Sample of Women: The Women's Cardiovascular Health Network Project* (ed: Amy A. Eyler) The Haworth Medical Press, an imprint of The Haworth Press, Inc., 2002, pp. 59-74. Single or multiple copies of this article are available for a fee from The Haworth Document Delivery Service [1-800-HAWORTH, 9:00 a.m. - 5:00 p.m. (EST). E-mail address: getinfo@haworthpressinc.com].

conducted with women aged 20 to 34 years and three with women aged 35 to 50 to evaluate response differences by age. Because no obvious age differences were observed, data were pooled. Barriers to physical activity included inadequate support for household and child care responsibilities and difficulties balancing home-related and societal expectations with physical activity. In addition, women reported little support from their communities and work sites to be physically active. Environmental barriers included lack of safe outdoor areas and accessible walking trails. Weather and stray dogs were also commonly mentioned. Sociocultural barriers included giving family obligations priority above all other things, being expected to eat large portions of high-fat foods, and failing to follow a traditionally active lifestyle. Enablers of physical activity included support from family and coworkers and participation in traditional community events. Suggested intervention approaches included accessible and affordable programs and facilities, community emphasis on physical activity, and programs that incorporated the needs of larger women and of families. Participants emphasized a preference for programs that were compatible with the role expectations of their families and communities, and they expressed the desire for acceptance and encouragement to be physically active from the family, the community, the worksite, and their tribal leaders. *[Article copies available for a fee from The Haworth Document Delivery Service: 1-800-HAWORTH. E-mail address: <getinfo@haworthpressinc. com> Website: <http://www.HaworthPress.com> © 2002 by The Haworth Press, Inc. All rights reserved.]*

KEYWORDS. American Indian, exercise, barriers, environment

PURPOSE

American Indian women have lower levels of reported physical activity, particularly when expressed as leisure-time physical activity (Welty et al., 1995; Ellis and Campos-Outcalt, 1994; MMWR, 1994; Brownson et al., 2000). Consistent with their high rates of physical inactivity, American Indians have rising rates of cardiovascular disease and type 2 diabetes (Welty et al., 1995; USDHHS 1996). Relatively few data are available on the determinants of physical activity in American Indian women. Identifying and understanding the multitude of factors that affect the ability of a woman to be regularly active is essential for designing culturally appropriate, gender-specific, and sustainable interventions to increase their physical activity rates and decrease their risks of chronic disease. To date, sociodemographic determinants of physical activity have been examined primarily, and the influence of sociocultural, environmental, and policy variables has received limited attention.

The purpose of the present study was to conduct focus group interviews exploring sociocultural, environmental, and policy-related determinants of physical activity among sedentary women from two southwest Pueblo American Indian tribes. A qualitative design was used to allow for an in-depth exploration of these determinants that may not have been achievable with a more structured survey.

This investigation was part of a larger collaborative multi-site study of the Women's Cardiovascular Health (WCH) Network funded by the Centers for Disease Control and Prevention. The reader is referred to Eyler et al. (2002) for a detailed description of the protocol development, data analyses, and the open-ended questions used in the focus groups.

METHODS

Thirty women (mean age = 37.4 ± 10.6 years) participated in this study. Subjects were recruited from two rural Southwest Pueblo reservation communities through local work sites, community health clinics, and written advertisements posted within the communities. Over 95% of all individuals living in these communities is American Indian. Interested women completed a screening questionnaire to establish that they had not been regularly active for at least 6 months before the recruitment period. Inactivity was defined as participating in moderate and vigorous activities less than 30 minutes per day, five days per week. The University of New Mexico Health Sciences Center Human Research and Review Committee and the institutional review board at the Centers for Disease Control and Prevention approved this study. In addition, permission was obtained from participating tribal agencies. Informed consent was obtained from all participants.

Data were collected during six focus group sessions conducted in the participating communities. Questions related to sociodemographic, psychological, sociocultural, environmental, and policy determinants of physical activity were posed. Because so much data were collected, the WCH Network agreed to limit this report to sociocultural, environmental, and policy factors. Three focus groups included women aged 20 to 35 years, and three were of women 36 to 50. A trained focus group moderator led each session with assistance from an American Indian co-moderator using methods recommended by Krueger and Casey (2000). Each session was audiotaped with permission of the participants, and the tapes were transcribed verbatim. Individuals were paid $10 for their participation.

Personal identifiers were removed as the transcripts were reviewed for accuracy; members of research staff compared the tape to the transcript, making corrections. Codes designated by the WCH Network researchers were applied. Two researchers independently coded each transcript, then met to agree on a common set of codes. Coded transcripts were entered into the NUD*IST software program (QSR, version 4). Text retrievals were performed for each of the primary topic areas identified in the focus group questions. Each set of text retrievals was reviewed, and the range of responses and emergent themes were identified using an inductive process.

RESULTS

A quantitative analysis of the demographic characteristics of the participants is reported in Eyler et al. (2002). In general, the 30 American Indian women in the present study were obese as defined by reference data from the Third National Health and Nutrition Examination Survey (NHANES III) (Flegal & Troiano, 2000), with a mean body mass index (BMI; weight in kilograms divided by height in meters squared) of 35.1. Two-thirds (66.7%) were employed full-time, 96.7% had completed high school, and 13.3% were college graduates. More than 50% had taken some technical or college courses. Because no obvious differences were found between the responses of the younger (20 to 35) and the older (36 to 50) groups, data from all focus groups were combined to derive the over-arching themes. A summary of these results is provided in Table 1.

Sociocultural Determinants

Women expressed difficulty in balancing their roles as homemaker, wage earner, and parent while incorporating physical activity in their daily lives. Most participants indicated a lack of support for chores and child care, which meant they had little time or energy for physical activity.

> I guess traditionally it's because . . . the woman is raised to be in the home. Her main focus is her home, clean the house, do whatever you do in the home . . . And the man is the one who is the outside person. So, I guess those of us that are raised traditionally–I know I was, but of course, when I moved away, a lot of things changed and that's the thing I found hard coming home because my grandmother didn't approve of a lot of the stuff that I was doing. So it kind of brought me back down to earth when I came back to <the Tribe> because all of the stuff that I did out in the city was not acceptable at <the Tribe>.

... that a lot of it [being inactive] is time management. A lot of women tend to do an excessive amount of work and then when they're all tired out ... it's like they want to just sit down and get ready for the next round or whatever might come up because in our lifestyles ... it's always come and go, do this, and some chores take a lot out of you . . . like, for instance, preparation for certain doings, culturally. The women are the major carriers of the work that gets done. And when they expend their energy, they're tired and worn out and they tend to just say, "Well, just in case something else comes up, I better just rest." And then it becomes a case of poor time management, poor management of putting your priorities, like your own needs first.

Although not a common observation, some participants stated that a partner or family member(s) provided strong social support for being active, which was viewed positively.

The other night out of the blue he [her husband] said, "Let's go walking." So he's been really good in that he comes out and I can't say no because I'm the one that's complaining [about her weight]. He brings up the suggestion. And now it's [the support] in the kids, too ... So, I think my husband has been real supportive ...

Overall, the participants expressed frustration with the lack of community support for physical activity. Women indicated that physical activity is not valued as a priority by the community, as illustrated by little support to maintain facilities, programs, and equipment. Some women stated that community members did not support others in being more physically active. In general, these women felt that others in the community were judging them or felt threatened by people who were physically active. Many women feared being ridiculed or pressured about breaking societal norms if they were to do something for themselves, and they seemed to want acceptance from the community to be physically active.

We'll see somebody walking. You stand at the window and you're visiting someone, "Wow, so and so is walking." You know, and then to me sometimes I think, "God, if I go for a walk, everybody's going to look out the window." "Wow, look there's <participant> walking" [laughter]. And it's like a little small town, you know, so ... when you start exercising, everybody's going to be talking about you.

Feeling support from the community seemed to be tied to an interest in being more active. In addition, community-based activities such as church, family gatherings, and cultural events were seen as enablers of physical activity.

TABLE 1. Factors Identified by American Indian Women that Relate to Physical Activity

Socio-Cultural Environment	Physical Environment & Policy
Social Support–Enablers • Partner or family member(s) provide strong social support • Church, family gatherings, and cultural events provide physical activity opportunities Social Support–Barriers • Inadequate support for chores and child care, resulting in little time or energy for physical activity • Difficulty balancing the demands of their role as a homemaker with social expectations while incorporating physical activity into daily life • Physical activity not valued as a top priority by community • Women feel others are judging them or feel threatened by people who are physically active • Fear of ridicule or pressure about breaking societal norms Cultural Characteristics & Comparison • Strong cultural emphasis on family responsibilities as top priority • Acceptance of larger body type • Demands related to participation in traditional cultural events • Social norms to eat large portions of high-fat foods • Failure to maintain active lifestyle of past generations • Lack of facilities and programs seen as a change in their cultural priorities • Participation in traditional dances and cultural events as ways to increase physical activity	Work Environment–Barriers • Lack of employer-supported programs and events • Brief lunch break not conducive to being active • Failure to maintain self-motivation when activities and programs are offered • General apathy regarding physical activity at work site Work Environment–Enablers • Active coworkers Community Environment–Barriers • Lack of paved roads, shoulders on sides of roads, and accessible walking trails • Weather–wind, blowing dust, heat • Lack of access to affordable and convenient facilities • Stray dogs, snakes, dangerous drivers on road, fear of break-ins at unattended homes

Many women said there were no differences between various ethnic groups in motivation for physical activity. In these cases, participants indicated that the choice to be physically active was up to each individual, and being Indian or non-Indian was not a primary determinant.

> I think generally it's all the same. There's inactive people and active people in every race.

> So it doesn't really matter whether you're a white woman or an Indian. It's basically where you live, if you have more access to certain things . . . if you're in the city, you have more access to a lot of [physical activity-related] things.

At the same time, these women stated they were less competitive about physical appearance than non-Hispanic white women and consequently felt less motivated to be active to please men.

> . . . we're not raised like you are in the white man's world, where your figure is important, your looks, and all that, nutrition and stuff. We're not raised like that on the reservation. And I found that out because I lived in California for 17 years and it's very competitive out there as opposed to on the reservation. We're not competitive here as to how your looks are or how to comb your hair, how you dress, how your shape is.

The sociocultural determinants identified were related to personal, community, and environmental issues. For instance, the strong sociocultural emphasis on family responsibilities was seen as a barrier to being physically active, as the woman's role as a caretaker takes precedence over everything else. Also, these American Indian women believed their culture was more accepting of a larger body type and much less competitive about physical appearance than the non-Hispanic white culture. Thus, participants stated they were less active because they were not pressured to lose weight and maintain a slim figure. The sociocultural importance of family can also serve as a motivation to exercise. Some women said they wanted to exercise to be alive and healthy to help support and care for their children and grandchildren.

> . . . I push myself because of my girls. I tell myself, "My girls are my everything." So for them I do what I need to do . . . such as taking care of myself and living for them because I want to be around for a long time to come to see them grow up to be women.

Another sociocultural issue that was viewed as both a barrier to physical activity and an enabler were the physical and time demands of participating in traditional cultural events in the community. These events are very time-consuming, as they involve a great deal of cooking, organizing, and preparing of foods and other items. The women expressed feelings of being overwhelmed during these events and being too tired to maintain a regular activity program. They also recognized, however, that these events are scheduled only occasionally, and that these responsibilities should really be a barrier only during the time of the event.

Women also stated, however, that participating in traditional cultural events was an enabler of physical activity. A great deal of physical work is involved in the traditional food preparations. The women in this study did not participate in the tribal dances that are also part of these events, but they agreed that traditional dancing was an enabler of physical activity for other women.

Another sociocultural issue that acted as a barrier was the emphasis on conforming to social norms of eating large portions of heavy, fatty foods such as fried foods and fatty meats. The women reported easy access to large portions of such foods, felt pressured to eat a lot to avoid being rude, and emphasized that community and family events revolved around preparing and eating food.

> Because the food—after you eat chili stew and—or, you know, what we fix for dinner. You don't have the energy [laughter] to go out, you know, but if you have a salad, you feel good about it and you say, "Oh well, I'm doing good now, I might as well go walking. You know, I can go walk to Grandma's and back and feel good." But after you eat the bread and the stew and whatever else, I'm so tired. You find yourself in front of the TV . . .

Women also recognized a failure of the current generations to follow the traditional patterns of eating and daily physical activities that were an integral part of their ancestors' lives. These women emphasized how their ancestors farmed, hunted, chopped wood, and hauled water to meet the needs of a rural life. Some women looked up to their mothers and grandmothers as role models, and they stressed the important role of culture and tradition in providing opportunities for physical activity. In addition, participants recognized that their access to motorized transportation, TV, and fast foods had led to low levels of physical activity, and this departure from a traditional lifestyle was viewed as unhealthy.

> And we don't even have to go hunting our food any more. We just go to the grocery store. We have all the foods that are accessible to us . . . more healthy foods. Yet, the foods that my grandparents ate must have been very healthy because, you know, they lived long lives . . . looking at fam-

ilies [now], starting with my aunts on my dad's side, they're all diabetic and they're not well . . .

When I think of this [physically active woman], I'm thinking of a long time ago, when the women had to do everything by hand. I mean, they just had to. They had to chop wood. They had to get their own water. They had to walk, like my mother. We lived on a high place. She had to walk down stairs to go hang out the laundry. They baked bread in their ovens all the time and she–every Friday or Saturday she was baking bread, a 25-pound bag of flour. So they had to, more or less, do these things. Now, the modern-day women, we have <a local store> [laughter]. She [my mother] provides the oven bread or tortillas and fry bread if we want. I got so, so spoiled with her. And we've got the automatic washers and dryers . . . I have a dryer and I have a clothesline right outside. I could go hang out my clothes but I don't want to.

Lack of facilities and programs was seen as a sociocultural and an environmental barrier to physical activity. Many women believed that their culture (and present communities) no longer prioritized physical activity. The lack of activity programs for children; the absence of equipment, facilities, and programs for adults; and the general sense that the community did not support physically active lifestyles for women were viewed by some women as negative changes in their culture.

I just think with us, as Native Americans, it's just the way our culture is. Everything is instilled in us as kids the way–what we believe as we grow up to be adults. Exercise or physical activity is not on the top of the list all the time. And that comes, you know, from school as well, like I said, because like now with the kids at the elementary school, they are spending 30 minutes I think once a week in PE [physical education] . . . because of another program . . . reading is important, but the way they structure the daily program, they put so much emphasis on reading and less on other things, and physical education being one of them was cut.

Environmental and Policy Issues

The primary physical barriers to physical activity were aspects of living in a rural environment: few or no paved roads, shoulders on the sides of roads, or accessible walking trails. The weather was another significant barrier. Strong winds, blinding dust, and excessive heat sometimes inhibited outdoor physical activity, and participants recognized that the community could benefit from the planting of grass and trees. In addition, one reservation community did not have adequate quantities of clean, safe drinking water in the summer, leading to problems with dehydration and not being able to bathe after physical activity.

> . . . the wind is a major factor out here. You don't even want to go outside some days just because the wind starts up. And then now, of course, it's summer. It gets extremely hot. And some of us have skin conditions. You can't afford to be out there too long. Otherwise, you're, you know, setting yourself up for skin cancer.

Lack of access to affordable and convenient physical activity facilities was an important community issue. Although there were some places to exercise indoors, many of the women felt they were not open at convenient times, were not staffed by qualified personnel, and did not offer regular programs. Some women stated the facilities were not open consistently. Some participants who recognized there were exercise facilities and opportunities close to home, however, pointed out that barriers prevented them from using them.

The work site was identified as an important location to support physical activity, but most women working outside the home expressed concerns about the lack of employer-supported programs and events. Many participants reported they were allowed only 30 minutes for lunch, which prevented their being active at that time. Some women worked at sites where activity programs had been in place but eventually cancelled because of unidentified circumstances. Another common theme was the failure to maintain self-motivation when physical activity opportunities arose at the work site.

> One of the ladies [at work] took it upon herself . . . to initiate a walking program during lunch. She . . . put out a nice memo and everything . . . "Would you please walk with me during lunch?" You know, "Are you interested?" . . . So I signed up . . . her and I were the only two the first day to go out and walk during lunch. Then the second day came, "Oh, I forgot my tennis shoes" [laughter] . . . And after that, we haven't been back out walking again. So . . . it's really hard . . . for me to keep on track.

There appeared to be a general feeling of apathy about physical activity at work, which was reported to influence participation rates for programs in that setting. When work sites offered occasional activities, women stated that getting people involved and motivated to participate was particularly challenging, and they recognized that this lack of interest contributed to the cancellation of some programs.

Active coworkers were often cited as enablers of physical activity, as these people served as role models and exerted indirect peer pressure that encouraged women to increase their physical activity levels.

When I was working, the people that I worked with in Albuquerque were very active. The majority of them were either at the gym during noon or in the morning . . . so I began like walking at lunch. You know, it was just because everybody else was doing it, kind of peer pressure.

A few women felt that offering free child care, either through the work site or the general community, would enable more women to be physically active. In contrast, many women thought that taking care of their children should remain their primary responsibility, and they would accept assistance only from other family members. These women gave the impression that they would not take advantage of child care provided by the work site or community, as they were not comfortable with having non-family members care for their children.

Most women expressed concerns about safety issues related to being physically active. Although only one participant shared her concerns about activity-related injuries, most agreed that the primary safety issue was aggressive stray dogs roaming in packs. Other safety concerns included snakes, dangerous drivers on dirt roads, and fear of break-ins if the women left their homes unattended.

Intervention Suggestions

Women had numerous suggestions for increasing physical activity opportunities in their communities (see Table 2). In general, they felt they needed role models and open community support to help them increase their activity. In addition, they strongly emphasized providing family-oriented activities, structured group activities with their peers, particularly walking programs, and programs that offered opportunities at fitness levels appropriate for themselves and others. They stressed the need for increasing access to convenient, affordable facilities and safe walking trails. Worksite suggestions included providing facilities and programs on site and assigning time for exercise during the work day. It was emphasized that community women should be involved in identifying physical activity priorities and interests.

DISCUSSION

As a sedentary lifestyle contributes significantly to increased risk for chronic diseases, we need to know why American Indian women do not regularly engage in moderate or vigorous physical activity. The focus group data we collected from physically inactive women who were members of two southwest Pueblo American Indian tribes represent an important contribution, as to date there is limited information on the sociocultural, environmental, and

TABLE 2. Physical Activity Intervention Suggestions from American Indian Women

Socio-Cultural	Physical	Policy
• Holistic life center for women that includes time management classes, stress management classes, relationship counseling, and other health promotion issues • Solicit women's input on type and level of physical activity desired and offer programs appropriate for women's fitness levels • Organize structured group activities for women and families • Schedule convenient times for exercise and physical activity events • Identify active community role models • Find ways to motivate people to be physically active by emphasizing self-care and conducting medical screens to identify health problems • Motivate parents to act as role models for their children • Start physical activity programs and messages at a young age	• Build a community fitness center • Provide a safe, comfortable environment for women to be active • Provide walking trails and landscaping that will reduce dust • Provide bike trails • Maintain an environment that promotes healthy behaviors, such as safe, clean water, no junk food, and accessible physical activity opportunities • Build a work site exercise facility with a shower	• Hire qualified exercise professionals at facilities • Get commitment from the community to maintain activity programs over a long-term period despite initial lack of participation or interest • Have employers require physical activities during the workday • Provide group activities at work, and provide adequate time for these activities such as a longer lunch break, during the lunch hour, or during/after work hours • Provide affordable or free health club memberships as an employee benefit • Provide incentives for physical activity such as waiving of entry fees for fun runs, child care, food, a fun environment, and cash • Encourage school policies for promoting more PE and other activities during the week

policy determinants of physical activity among inactive American Indian women.

The participants described a multitude of issues that affected their ability to be physically active, with one overarching theme the great social and cultural pressure to conform to their roles as mothers and caretakers. As they tried to meet societal expectations, the women were not encouraged to take care of themselves as well, and they found it difficult to add regular physical activity to their work and home responsibilities. Similarly, Wilcox et al. (2000) used telephone interviews with rural women (including American Indians) and found that caregiver duties were most often cited as a barrier to physical activity. In-depth interviews of older American Indian women (mean age = 56 years) also emphasized the predominance of caregiving duties as an ingrained sociocultural expectation (Henderson & Ainsworth, 2000). These expectations appear to be an issue for all women, however; they are not unique to American Indian women (Henderson et al., 1996). An important finding of the present study was that participants did not express the desire to change societal norms, appearing more interested in finding strategies for increasing physical activity that were compatible with the role expectations of their families and communities. Family-oriented and community-supported activities were both suggested as compatible with societal norms. This is vital information that intervention specialists and policy makers can use in designing physical activity programs for these communities.

Participants in the present study indicated that a physically active lifestyle was not a priority in their communities. Many women felt they would be ridiculed or socially ostracized if they were seen exercising. The lack of support from family and community led to their feeling tired and stressed, which discouraged them from being active. Other studies of American Indian women have shown that those with less social support are not as active as those with more support (Eyler et al., 1999; Wilcox et al., 2000). Lack of time and energy and being too tired are also commonly reported barriers to physical activity in American Indian women, similar to other groups of women (Heesch et al., 2000; Wilcox et al., 2000; Henderson et al., 1999; Harnack et al., 1999a,b).

Other important sociocultural themes included the acceptance of a larger figure, expectations of eating large quantities of high-fat foods, and the lack of emphasis on physical activity among young children. Although some felt uncomfortable with being overweight, many believed that being overweight was culturally acceptable and encouraged. This social acceptance of a fuller figure could have important implications for the design and marketing of physical activity programs, as focusing on weight loss may be inappropriate and ineffective for many American Indian women. Notably, women in this study did not mention weight loss as a reason to be active. Their primary reasons to be physically active included feeling better, treatment for their illnesses (e.g., diabetes), and prolonging their lives (data not included). These are important findings, as no similar data were found in previously studies of this population. If confirmed in a larger sample of American Indian women, these findings should prove important in designing culturally appropriate interventions for this population.

Limited resources and facilities and failure to maintain programs over long periods of time were seen as challenges to being physically active. In an earlier study, Henderson and Ainsworth (2000) found that limited resources acted as a barrier to physical activity for American Indian women more than for African

American women. Women in the present study also expressed a need for facilities and programs that were designed specifically for large women, and they suggested incorporating programs for time management, stress reduction, and other areas of health promotion. The biggest safety issue was loose, aggressive dogs, a common concern among American Indian women in rural settings (Wilcox et al., 2000; Harnack et al., 1999b; Stolarczyk et al., 1999).

Participants reminisced about the highly active lifestyles of their older relatives and earlier ancestors, and they viewed low levels of physical activity as negative changes in their social and cultural environment. Henderson et al. (1999) and Henderson and Ainsworth (2000) also emphasized the importance of the cultural context of physical activity for American Indian women.

The participants in the present study shared numerous ideas regarding interventions that could increase their physical activity levels. Providing affordable and convenient facilities and programs was one approach; another was designing programs that include families, which may be seen as more socially acceptable than having women exercise while their children are in day care. Programs also must be designed to meet specific needs and concerns, without being seen as threatening to family and societal norms. Emphasis on weight loss would most likely be ineffective in increasing physical activity in these women; it may be more appropriate to emphasize how the health of families and communities is strengthened by regular physical activity. Although there is not a simple solution to the presence of dangerous dogs, providing access to more indoor activities and outdoor group programs may help eliminate this barrier for some women.

One of the major limitations of the present study is that these results were not gathered from a large number of culturally diverse tribal members, being obtained from two Pueblo communities. As there are 556 federally recognized American Indian tribes in the contiguous 48 states (Bureau of Indian Affairs, 2000), our results are not representative of all American Indian women. A second limitation is that these data represent the opinions of women who were both sedentary and willing and able to volunteer for this study. Physically active women would likely have identified or emphasized factors other than those presented in this paper. Despite these limitations, this study makes an important contribution to the limited but expanding literature addressing determinants of physical activity among American Indian women.

CONCLUSIONS

There is no one intervention that can increase physical activity levels for all women in a community. Encouraging tribal leaders to publicly make physical activity a top health priority will send a strong message that may motivate communities to increase their physical activity levels. In contrast, recommendations from the U.S. government for changing health behavior seem relatively ineffective in these communities, most likely because of the historically difficult relationships between tribes and the federal government. Researchers, tribal leaders, community members, and work site supervisors need to jointly implement a variety of programs and opportunities to increase regular physical activity. It is imperative, however, that the community members who will be directly affected by facilities and programs be included in the planning, implementation, and evaluation of physical activity interventions. By assessing women's needs and working directly with communities, we increase our potential for designing culture- and gender-appropriate physical activity programs that can be sustained.

REFERENCES

Brownson, R.C., Eyler, A.A., King, A.C., Brown, D.R., Shyu, Y.L., & Sallis, J.F. (2000). Patterns and correlates of physical activity among US women 40 years and older. *American Journal of Public Health 90* (2), 264-270.

Bureau of Indian Affairs. (2000). *List of federally recognized American Indian tribes and Alaska Natives. <http://www.doi.gov/bia/tribes/entry.html>*.

Centers for Disease Control and Prevention. (1997). Monthly estimates of leisure-time physical inactivity–United States, 1994. *Morbidity and Mortality Weekly Report 46* (18), 393-397.

Ellis, J.L., & Campos-Outcalt, D. (1994). Cardiovascular disease risk factors in Native Americans: A literature review. *American Journal of Preventive Medicine 10* (5), 295-307.

Eyler, A.A., Brownson, R.C., Donatelle, R.J., King, A.C., Brown, D., & Sallis, J.F. (1999). Physical activity social support and middle- and older-aged minority women: Results from a US survey. *Social Science & Medicine 49* (6), 781-789.

Flegal, K.M., & Troiano, R.P. (2000). Changes in the distribution of body mass index of adults and children in the US population. *International Journal of Obesity and Related Metabolic Disorders 24* (7), 807-818.

Harnack, L., Sherwood, N., & Story, M. (1999a). Diet and physical activity patterns of urban American Indian women. *American Journal of Health Promotion 13* (4), 233-236.

Harnack, L., Story, M., & Holy Rock, B. (1999b). Diet and physical activity patterns of Lakota Indian adults. *Journal of the American Dietetic Association 99* (7), 829-835.

Heesch, K.C., Brown, D.R., & Blanton, C.J. (2000). Perceived barriers to exercise and stage of exercise adoption in older women of different racial/ethnic groups. *Women & Health 30* (4), 61-76.

Henderson, K.A., & Ainsworth, B.E. (2000). Enablers and constraints to walking for older African American and American Indian women: The Cultural Activity Participation Study. *Research Quarterly for Exercise and Sport 71* (4), 313-321.

Henderson, K.A., Ainsworth, B.E., Stolarzcyk, L.M., Hootman, J.M., & Levin, S. (1999). Notes on linking qualitative and quantitative data: The Cross Cultural Physical Activity Participation Study. *Leisure Sciences 21*(3), 247-255.

Henderson, K.A., Bialschki, M.D., Shaw, S.M., & Frevsinger, V.J. 1996. *Both gains and gaps.* State College, PA: Venture Publishing, Inc.

Krueger, R.A., & Casey, M.A. (2000). *Focus Groups. A practical guide for applied research.* 3rd Edition. Thousand Oaks, CA: Sage Publications, Inc.

Stolarczyk, L.M., Gilliland, S.S., Lium, D.J., Owen, C.L., Perez, G.E., Kriska, A.M., Ainsworth, B.E., & Carter, J.S. (1999). Knowledge, attitudes and behaviors related to physical activity among Native Americans with diabetes. *Ethnicity & Disease 9* (1), 59-69.

Indian Health Service. (1996). *Trends in Indian Health.* Rockville, MD: US Department of Health and Human Services, Public Health Service, Indian Health Services.

Welty, T.K., Lee, E.T., Yeh, J., Cowan, L.D., Go, O., Fabsitz, R.R., Le, N.A., Oopik, A.J., Robbins, D.C., & Howard, B.V. (1995). Cardiovascular disease risk factors among American Indians: The Strong Heart Study. *American Journal of Epidemiology 142* (3), 269-287.

Wilcox, S., Castro, C., King, A.C., Housemann, R., & Brownson, R.C. (2000). Determinants of leisure time physical activity in rural compared with urban older and ethnically diverse women in the United States. *Journal of Epidemiology and Community Health 54* (9), 667-672.

Environmental, Policy, and Cultural Factors Related to Physical Activity Among Rural, African American Women

Bonnie Sanderson, PhD, RN
MaryAnn Littleton, PhD
LeaVonne Pulley, PhD

SUMMARY. Sixty-one African American women (ages 20-50 years) from a rural community in Alabama participated in six focus groups. Barriers to and enablers of physical activity were identified and grouped into personal, environmental (social and physical), policy, and cultural themes for qualitative analyses. Personal factors included motivation, perceived health, feeling tired, and lack of time; social environmental

Bonnie Sanderson is affiliated with the University of Alabama at Birmingham, Birmingham, AL 35294. MaryAnn Littleton and LeaVonne Pulley are affiliated with the Department of Health Behavior, School of Public Health, Ryals Public Health Building, University of Alabama at Birmingham, Birmingham, AL 35294.

Address correspondence to: Bonnie Sanderson, PhD, RN, University of Alabama at Birmingham, 307 LHRB, 701 19th Street South, Birmingham, AL 35294 (E-mail: bsanderson@uabmc.edu).

The authors thank Stacey Shelton for her assistance with this project and the preparation of the manuscript. The authors also gratefully thank Ethel Mixon-Johnson and Janice Ward for their assistance with this project and all the women of Wilcox County who participated in the focus groups.

This research was supported by a grant from the Robert Wood Johnson Foundation (I.D. # 038325) in collaboration with centers funded from the Centers for Disease Control and Prevention, Special Interest Project # 5.

[Haworth co-indexing entry note]: "Environmental, Policy, and Cultural Factors Related to Physical Activity Among Rural, African American Women." Sanderson, Bonnie, MaryAnn Littleton, and LeaVonne Pulley. Co-published simultaneously in *Women & Health* (The Haworth Medical Press, an imprint of The Haworth Press, Inc.) Vol. 36, No. 2, 2002, pp. 75-90; and: *Environmental, Policy, and Cultural Factors Related to Physical Activity in a Diverse Sample of Women: The Women's Cardiovascular Health Network Project* (ed: Amy A. Eyler) The Haworth Medical Press, an imprint of The Haworth Press, Inc., 2002, pp. 75-90. Single or multiple copies of this article are available for a fee from The Haworth Document Delivery Service [1-800-HAWORTH, 9:00 a.m. - 5:00 p.m. (EST). E-mail address: getinfo@haworthpressinc.com].

factors included support from friends, family, and issues related to child care; physical environmental factors included weather, access to facilities, availability of sidewalks or other places to walk; policy factors included personal safety concerns (loose dogs, traffic, etc.) and inflexible work environments. Some, but not all, women perceived cultural differences as a factor affecting physical activity levels. Differences in socioeconomic levels and time demands among women of different cultures were identified as factors that may influence physical activity. Participants provided suggestions for community-based physical activity interventions using an environmental approach. *[Article copies available for a fee from The Haworth Document Delivery Service: 1-800-HAWORTH. E-mail address: <getinfo@haworthpressinc.com> Website: <http://www.HaworthPress. com> © 2002 by The Haworth Press, Inc. All rights reserved.]*

KEYWORDS. Physical activity, women's health, African American/ Black, rural, community health

PURPOSE

African American women are at special risk for physical inactivity (DDHS, 1996; Brownson, Eyler, King, Brown, Shyu, & Sallis, 2000) and rural, southern regions of the United States report some of the highest rates of physical inactivity (Centers for Disease Control and Prevention [CDC], 1998; Duelburg, 1992). The prevalence of physical inactivity is specially burdensome in Alabama, where 83% of African Americans and 78% of whites were found (by self-report) to engage in less than 30 minutes of moderate intensity activity 5 days a week (CDC, 1998; Phillips & Cook, 2001). The purpose of this article is to report the findings from focus groups that explored rural African American women's perceptions about physical activity. Although we explored a wide range of factors that may affect physical activity behaviors, our specific focus was to explore environmental and cultural issues that may be unique among rural African American women.

The sample included adult African American women (aged 20-50 years) residing in a rural community in Wilcox County in southwest Alabama. Of a county population of some 13,500, 70% are African American, and 40% live below the poverty level (DDHS, Community Health Status Report, 2000). Participants were recruited by a community-based project coordinator who placed ads in the local newspaper, distributed flyers to public places (e.g., grocery stores, churches), and spread the word through community contacts. The project coordinator screened interested women by telephone and scheduled those eligible for age-specific focus groups (20-35 or 36-50 years). Eligibility criteria included being an African American woman residing in the Wilcox County area and currently (during the past 6 months) not exercising regularly (three times a week for at least 20 minutes). To explore enablers of and barriers to physical activity among women of various cultures, the major themes included personal (biological and psychological), environmental (social and physical), policy, and cultural factors that may affect physical activity behavior.

Six focus groups were conducted in May 2000 in a community center in Wilcox County. Three groups included women aged 20-35 years and three included women aged 36-50 years. Women received a cash incentive of $20. An experienced moderator facilitated each focus group, with each session audio-recorded while a trained assistant manually took notes. Each participant signed an informed consent and completed a brief paper-and-pencil demographic questionnaire. The audiotapes were transcribed verbatim and coded using QSR NUD*IST®, which is a qualitative software program that uses non-numerical unstructured data for indexing searching and theory-building (Sage, 1996). The transcribed data were scanned in sections for words and phrases that related to the concepts and themes of interest and assigned the appropriate codes using this program.

RESULTS

A total of 61 women (mean age, 36 yrs ± 8.4) attended the focus groups, with 26 women (mean age, 28 yrs ± 5.1) attending the younger group and 35 (mean, 41 yrs ± 5.2) the middle-aged groups. Because of the similarity of results of the two sets of groups, we combined them in this report, with specific notations when group differences were found. Most participants were employed (85%), had some education past high school (67%), and were not married (66%). The majority of women were obese (66%), perceived their health as good or very good (77%), and reported low physical activity during both work (63%) and non-work (56%) hours.

Our network project adopted categorical themes that helped the focus group moderators explore barriers to and enablers of physical activity among women of various cultures: (1) personal (biological and psychological), (2) environmental (social and physical), (3) policy, and (4) cultural. We describe our findings for these themes, then summarize the participants' suggestions for interventions to promote physical activity.

Personal (Biological and Psychological)

Being too physically tired to exercise, especially because of demanding work and family schedules, emerged as a major barrier. Middle-aged women mentioned that being overweight also prevented physical activity by making them tired and unmotivated. Poor health was also mentioned as a deterrent. Statements expressing these points of view include the following:

> When you get to work you are too tired from getting up in the morning and fussing with the kids to get out of the car for day care. When you get to work, you just work . . . by lunchtime you're hungry . . . you eat and you try to start one more time . . . And when you get home you got to cook, clean up, wash clothes . . . you're just too tired.

> Mine is my weight . . . it's just my weight. I feel tired, I try but still I just can't go sometimes.

> You know, I guess it's my health. One time I was involved in exercise class and everything, but then I got ill . . . since I've been back up again, I don't exercise, period.

In contrast, one woman who said, "It's easier to exercise because you know you are supposed to do it," described her medical condition as an enabler. Another woman mentioned body weight as an enabler by saying, "The lighter you are the more you want to go."

Some major psychological barriers expressed included time issues, choices on spending discretionary time, not enjoying physical activity, not knowing about the "right" physical activity, and various other motivational issues.

Statements relating to personal barriers included the following:

> By the time I get home I have to take care of them (children) . . . It makes it hard for me because I don't have much time for myself. I don't have time for exercise without them.

> Television, had it not been invented, maybe I would have more hours in the day.

> Well, there are really no excuses for me . . . I just don't take the time.

> Exercising by yourself is boring . . .

> Not having anything interesting to do . . .

> Not knowing the type of exercises to fit you . . .

> Where I work, it's easy because when I have my break, I could go and walk around the gym . . . I'm just being lazy.

It doesn't have anything to do with how we work or what we do, it's just the state of mind, we're just not motivated to do it because we're not used to doing it.

Comments concerning positive motivating factors included being active as a stimulus for more activity, liking your job, and being concerned with your appearance when you are sexually active:

The more you exercise the more energy you have and you can last longer.

The more you move, the more you can . . .

If you like your job, it helps. You have to like your job first. If I like my job, I'm ready to get up and go. It makes me real motivated.

The appearance of their bodies . . . you know, they concentrate on that more when they are sexually active . . . they worry about how they are going to look, you know, when they take their clothes off.

Social Environment

The main issues relating to the social environment included support from family, friends, neighbors, and the neighborhood. Children were seen as both an enabler and a barrier. They were enablers because taking care of children requires physical activity in just "keeping up with them" and because children engage in physical play more often than adults, they often encourage adults to play sports or games with them. Younger women mentioned that taking children with them when they walk or having cooperative children allowed them time to walk or go to an aerobics class.

In contrast, the presence of children was perceived to be a barrier when childcare issues prevented women from independently exercising or getting involved in structured exercise programs. Specific comments related to childcare issues included the following:

Sometimes, when you can find a baby sitter, you don't do anything, because you are so used to having them there with you. You are so lost without them, and then when you have them there, they drive you crazy (so) you can't exercise.

I think the main thing is that you want to exercise but you just can't because nobody will keep them (children) for you . . .

> If they've kept your child all day so you can work, you don't want to ask them to keep them all evening because you want to respect their time, they may have something they want to do.

> When you say, "Can you keep the kids while I go exercise?" People say you don't need to do that.

> That's the main thing, child care, and if you have somebody, you want to make sure they get fed and taken care of . . . but everybody is not going to treat your kids like you treat them, and it can be you own relatives . . . child care, that's the main thing.

Other influences included hot weather, competing social activities, being around others who were overweight, and not being motivated.

> I am not going out in the hot sun . . . then you say you are going to wait until it gets cooler to go out and exercise . . . but someone asks you to go play cards . . . wants to go to some other place . . . (then) you are going to forget all about (exercise) and go play cards!

> The people I live with are overweight and not motivated, which makes it harder . . .

The social aspects of neighbors and neighborhoods and observing others being active in the neighborhood seemed to influence physical activity among some women.

> Well, no one else in the neighborhood is active . . . that's hard. If you see someone else out there, that would motivate you to get out there with them.

> I do not socialize with my neighbors . . . I have one neighbor I socialize with . . . and then my mother. If you don't participate into the things they are into, well, they always look at you funny. And you know to keep down (this) feeling, I stay on my own, I stay in my own house.

The women did mention negative influences from the social environment and described some discouraging or negative remarks they heard when they were engaged in outdoor physical activity. Such comments as "people hollering at you," "whistling, making jokes," "following you in the car" or "drivebys" alluding to feelings of personal safety threats when exercising outdoors. In addition, specific comments linking physical activity and body weight evoked negative feelings, such as "She needs to go home with her fat self" or "You ain't gonna lose no weight, so go home."

In contrast, some statements reflected positive feelings about neighbors and neighborhoods seeming to increase a feeling of safety when exercising outdoors:

> We have good neighbors and you can walk anytime you want to, and there are no thieves around . . . we've got a good neighborhood.

> Everybody looks out for everybody . . .

Ironically, a negative comment about the neighborhood took on a positive twist for a woman who lived near a park where litter was a problem:

> . . . you know you got a nasty neighborhood, then the wind blows, and the paper comes in your yard. Then you have to pick up other people's paper . . . well, I've got to go get it out of the yard . . . it helps me get it (physical activity).

Physical Environment

Hot weather and the lack of safe places to walk were frequently mentioned as barriers. Conversely, the quiet, rural area and low-traffic country roads were seen as encouraging to walkers.

Both lack of facilities and being too far from facilities were cited as barriers. No community or recreational centers with exercise equipment were identified and sidewalks, streetlights, and parks were scarce. Parks that were available were mostly seen as poorly equipped or inadequately maintained. The community high school was identified as having a swimming pool that was accessible in the summer and it offered a water aerobics class. Some women expressed concerns about safety and adequate supervision of this pool. A physical therapy center was cited as an exercise resource the community could use but others said the area was too small and the fees were expensive for general exercise use. The cost of fitness facilities or programs emerged as a barrier to physical activity:

> It's just the income; the resources are not available. When I say the resources, I mean if I had the resources I could get involved. The more resources, the more money, the more motivated . . . at least I am . . . Not saying that money is the controller of life, but I'm realistic.

Walking was frequently discussed as a favorable physical activity. Many women identified "the best place for walking" as the high school parking lot, but it was not convenient for some. Participants mentioned that some neighborhoods were relatively more convenient for walking and also "helped you go to where you needed to go."

Policy

Work environments were usually perceived as barriers. Comments were made about not having a long enough lunch break to allow walking, or of day care centers closing early. One woman vented her feelings about her employer's lack of encouragement by saying, "They encourage you to work more, and that's it." Some women did mention ways to increase physical activity during the workday, such as using the stairs, walking instead of riding, and walking during breaks.

Major safety concerns related to walking were the lack of sidewalks, streetlights, and the presence of unleashed or stray dogs that bothered people. Some areas had speed breakers for traffic, and some apparently had residents who were better at keeping their dogs fenced. One younger woman described her concern about violence:

> A safe neighborhood . . . (needs to) cut down some of the violence. (A woman) . . . doesn't want to go outside . . . Thugs . . . you don't ever know when there's going to be a driveby . . . you be too scared to walk.

Culture

Cultural issues emerged as potential factors among some, but not all women. Some perceived that African American women had less socioeconomic resources than Caucasians, with the African Americans working harder at jobs with less pay and not being able to afford baby sitters or memberships to exercise facilities. They also perceived their jobs as more physically demanding than those of Caucasians, which led to different patterns of physical activity than that group. Overlapping themes of work, family, and household responsibilities causing fatigue and limiting time and resources to be physically active were sounded repeatedly. Frequently, these factors were expressed as contributing to a larger burden to African American women than those of different cultures, especially Caucasian women. Several statements articulated these perceptions:

> We have to do all the work ourselves and them other folks can hire someone to do it for them; because of money, we don't have the availability to money, a baby-sitter, you know, we need to take care of those kids.

One thing different . . . it appears to me that they (whites) are more physically active than we are . . . and I notice that the barriers might be that we don't have the money to join the exercise place whereas they might have it, financial wise.

I think there are differences in ways that they get their physical activity. Because I think that black women work hard, and that is just my opinion. I think black as a race, African American or whatever, they work harder than Caucasians (whites) . . . go back and think about it . . . who is actually working the hardest? No matter what the job is, and I work several, it looks like I did most of the work . . .

The lack of physically active female role models was also mentioned as a potential cultural difference between African American women and other cultural groups. One woman described her culture as not seeing women exercising, but instead seeing the number one priority for women as taking care of their home and family. This theme also surfaced when women described the competing responsibilities of work and family, which did not allow time for structured physical activity:

Because I think it is the way they are raised. I think Caucasian women are brought up in a household where their mothers, or their aunt, or whoever, are physically active when they were growing up, so it was kind of put on them. But when you are an African American, Asian, or whatever, the mothers are usually hardworking . . . they do not have time. Just like everyone was saying they have to come home and cook and clean. They do not have time for physical activity, therefore, when you are growing up you don't think, "I need to exercise, but, I need to do this and I need to do that," because it (physical activity) is not done around you.

Views on body image emerged as another perceived cultural difference between African American and Caucasian women:

. . . most black women don't worry a whole lot about their body . . . they are big, they like hips . . . they don't see it as a big problem for that kind of a body shape; white men . . . if they (women) are not thin, there's something wrong with them. But with us, we kind of like it.

Caucasians . . . they are obsessed with being thin, you know, but with African Americans it's a slight compliment to you, the heavier you are, it is more acceptable in the African American community.

Despite the comments on cultural differences, there were women in both age groups who hesitated to conclude that differences in physical activity patterns were related to culture:

> I guess it depends on the person, they just want to do it . . .

> Well you know, lots of people are brought up different ways, a lot of people exercise because they are used to doing it.

> Yeah, it's a personal thing I don't think it's got anything to do with cultures, it's a personal thing.

> Different people just believe in different things, it's not because of the cultural background . . .

There were some perceptions that women in the African American culture were less likely to choose being active compared to women from other cultures:

> A lot of them (whites) have the same jobs we have . . . they have to do the same duties we do when they get off work, but they make that lunch break valuable. They walk on their lunch break.

> African Americans don't put food down for nothing. Eating and sleeping, then you eat so much and you're so full. Walk? Huh . . . It's too hot out there, girl!

> I have some friends who are Chinese. They are very active, they always stay on the go. They are always doing things, even if it is just in the house or out in the yard. They are always doing something in the yard, whereas I would go home, I wouldn't be out fixing my flowerbed . . . that is every day for them. I might go inside and cook and clean . . . then I am going to sit down and rest. She (Chinese woman) is never going to sit down and rest, she is always thinking of something to do. All the time.

One woman expressed a difference between rural and urban black women in that urban women may be more active because, "Some of the urban black women tend to take more pride in it, I guess. Even if they don't follow through with it, they still try to do it."

Table 1 summarizes the factors identified in the focus groups as enablers and barriers to physical activity among these rural, African American women.

TABLE 1. Factors Identified as Enablers and Barriers to Physical Activity Among Rural, African-American Women

Socio-Cultural Environment	Physical Environment and Policy
Social Support	Physical Environment and Policy Issues
Enablers and Barriers • Support from family, friends, neighbors • Children; childcare Barriers • Competing activities–home, work, and social • Being around other people who are not active or motivated • Verbal insults when attempting to be active outside Cultural Comparisons • Individual motivation was frequently perceived as more important than cultural influences When cultural differences were expressed, African-Americans were perceived as having: • Less resources (time and money) for physical activity • Fewer physically active role models • More physically demanding jobs • Less obsession with "thinness" • Different choices when spending discretionary time	Enablers • Safe and convenient places to exercise • Quiet, low-traffic country roads • Good neighborhood Barriers • Hot weather • Negative or discouraging remarks from others • Poorly maintained or equipped parks or recreational grounds • Fast-driving traffic, especially trucks • Unleashed dogs • Threat to personal safety • Work environments not flexible • Lack of sidewalks, streetlights • Lack of facilities, or too far away or costly

Interventions

The final question posed to the participants was, "If you were a community leader with unlimited funds, what would you do to promote physical activity in your community?" This prompted active discussion from all groups and generated suggestions for interventions using environmental approaches that may be effective in increasing physical activity among rural African American women. The following suggestions are illustrated in Table 2 and briefly summarized here.

Social Environment

To enhance the social environment, participants suggested offering group exercise classes or recreational programs on a regular basis. They also sug-

TABLE 2. Physical Activity Interventions: Suggestions from Rural, African-American Women

Socio-Cultural Environment	Physical Environment	Policy
• Provide educational classes on healthy lifestyles, diet and physical activity • Promote physical activity through motivational speakers, articles, flyers • Organize a marathon or walk/run races Provide exercise classes and/or programs: • Aerobics • Tennis • Swimming • Exercise equipment • Bowling • Skating • Dance, Taebo • Volleyball Organize childcare activities • Childcare cooperative (trade childcare services) • Tutoring program for older children Organize group physical activity opportunities • Walking clubs • Exercise classes or programs at churches • Community ball teams (softball, basketball, little league, etc.)	Build opportunities for pleasant walking experiences • More sidewalks–inside and outside of city limits • Walking and bicycle trails • Shopping mall Build a recreational or community center which includes specialty areas, programs: • Swimming Pool • Tennis Courts • Sport Gym • Exercise Gym • Childcare Center • Teen Center • Senior Citizen Create an outdoor family activity area • Walking track or trail • Playground area in the center of the track/trail for children • Include playground equipment for children Build sport areas • Ball Fields • Golf Course	• Improve and/or install lighting in parks and streets • Improve up-keep and cleanliness of community and recreational grounds, including parks (broken glass, wooded areas) • Extend hours at work for childcare • Provide childcare at no cost for low income mothers • Provide transportation for the elderly or those without transportation to a community or recreational center • Provide at-work exercise programs • Create more jobs in the community that increase financial resources • Provide experienced, competent lifeguards at swimming pool • Remove or control all loose or stray dogs

gested organizing walking clubs or ball teams within already established groups such as church congregations or fellow employees. It was clearly expressed that childcare would have to be included if women were expected to participate in such group activities.

Physical Environment

Building structures and facilities that would accommodate more physical activities were suggested by several women; no women knew of a community recreational center available for group exercise classes. Participants also voiced a need for improving outdoor areas that would promote pleasant walking experiences, such as sidewalks, walking and bicycle trails, ball fields, and playground areas with safe equipment. One woman suggested creating a walking track and placing a playground area in the center so that children could play while their mothers walked for exercise. This would allow a safe way for them to be active and together.

Policy

Participants suggested better maintenance of community grounds and parks, improved lighting in public areas, having experienced lifeguards for swimming programs, and enforced control of loose dogs. They also suggested that work sites could provide onsite exercise programs and that childcare centers should extend their hours of operation to make it more convenient for women to exercise after work. Providing transportation to elderly residents or others with special needs was also mentioned to increase access to physical activity programs in this rural community.

DISCUSSION

These focus groups produced some interesting results concerning perceived barriers to physical activity among rural African American women as well as tactics to enhance such activity. There is a paucity of literature on physical activity in rural populations in general and rural African American women in particular. The information should be especially useful in developing effective interventions for African American women living in rural areas. To date, most studies that have explored correlates of physical activity focused primarily on personal or sociodemographic factors (Eyler et al., 2001). However, more recent reports (Wilcox, Castro, King, Housemann, & Brownson, 2000; King, Castro, Wilcox, Eyler, Sallis, & Brownson, 2000) have described some important environmental factors associated with physical activity behaviors among women of different ethnic groups. The unique aspect of the present study was its comprehensive exploration of a wide spectrum of determinants of physical activity, including psychosocial, environmental and policy, and cultural factors.

Most personal factors we identified as perceived barriers were similar to those findings found in other studies (Wilcox et al., 2000; Eyler, Baker, Cromer, King, Brownson, & Donatelle, 1998). Specifically, we identified perceived lack of time, social support, motivation, and child care responsibilities. We note that care-giving duties were identified as major barriers to leisure-time physical activity among rural African American women in an earlier report (Wilcox et al., 2000), and health concerns were reported to be a barrier to physical activity among African American women in another study (Eyler et al., 1998). We found mixed results, however, concerning health issues. Some women considered poor health as a barrier and yet some women perceived a health condition an enabler if they thought physical activity would improve their health. This finding may have important implications for health care professionals in guiding their patients with health concerns regarding physical activity.

As in other studies (Wilcox et al., 2000; Eyler et al., 1998; Eyler, Brownson, Donatell, Brown, & Sallis, 1999), social support was perceived to be an important factor. Our study emphasized the added importance of support in issues related to child care such as feeling comfortable when asking for help, having quality care available, or having options for extended hours in day care facilities that would make it more convenient to exercise. The findings in this study also highlighted a negative influence in the social environment involving verbal remarks commonly heard by women attempting to walk in some neighborhoods of Wilcox County, Alabama. Having a safe, supportive environment in which to be physically active seems an important issue to address in rural communities.

Most women thought the physical environment was an important influence on physical activity behaviors. Participants readily identified the lack of facilities, or nearby facilities, or areas that were poorly equipped or maintained as negative influences. As in another report (Eyler et al., 1998), access to programs and the cost of programs were viewed as deterrents to structured exercise. With respect to the natural environment, the hot Alabama weather was seen as a negative influence. Other concerns included safety issues such as unleashed or stray dogs. Some women perceived pleasant surroundings such as quiet country roads as a positive influence, which recalls other studies (Wilcox et al., 2000; King et al., 2000) that reported similar effects from pleasant scenery. Walking was seen as a favorable and viable option for most of these focus group participants if there were safe, convenient, and pleasant areas to walk. This finding is similar to other studies that reported physical activity behavior in community settings (Brownson et al., 2000; King et al., 2000; Siegel, Brackbill, & Heath, 1995).

Cultural issues affecting physical activity among various ethnic/culture groups have rarely been explored in research settings. Our findings produced mixed results concerning the impact of culture on physical activity behaviors. Some women expressed beliefs that African American women were at a disadvantage for being physically active due to deficient financial resources, a lack of social support, and few physically active role models. Some women also expressed different values placed on body image or size when comparing the African American culture with other cultures, especially to the Caucasian culture.

Other women, however, perceived that culture was not a major influence and that physical activity was more of a personal choice. More research is needed related to cultural influences on physical activity behaviors, especially among more sedentary populations.

CONCLUSION

This study increases our knowledge and understanding of physical activity behaviors and some perceived barriers and enablers to physical activity among rural African American women. By exploring personal, environmental, policy, and cultural factors, we were able to expand our understanding of the multidimensional influences that may affect physical activity behaviors in a community setting. The qualitative analysis provides some valuable information in developing in-depth quantitative research exploring physical activity behaviors among African American women, a group at high risk for physical inactivity. Furthermore, the information gained will provide insight to public health professionals for planning community-based interventions that include effective environmental approaches to promote and maintain a physically active community.

REFERENCES

Brownson, R.C., Eyler, A.A., King, A.C., Brown, D.R., Shyu, Y.L., Sallis, J.F. (2000). Patterns and correlates of physical activity among US women 40 years and older. *American Journal of Public Health*, 90(2), 264-270.

Centers for Disease Control and Prevention. (1998). Behavioral Risk Surveillance System. Survey data, 1998. Atlanta, GA: United States Department of Health and Human Services, National Center for Chronic Disease Prevention and Health Promotion. http://www.cdc.gov/nccdphp/brfss/. Accessed February 20, 2001.

Centers for Disease Control and Prevention. (1998). Self-reported physical inactivity by degree of urbanization: United States, 1996. *Morbidity and Mortality Weekly Report*, 47(50), 1097-1100.

U.S. Department of Health and Human Services. (2000). *Health Resources and Services Administration. Community Health Status Report: Wilcox County, Ala, July 2000.* <http://www.communityhealth.gov>. Accessed January 10, 2001.

U.S. Department of Health and Human Services. (1996). *Physical Activity and Health: A report of the Surgeon General.* Atlanta, GA: Centers for Disease Control and Prevention, National Center for Chronic Disease Prevention and Health Promotion.

Duelberg, S.I. (1992). Preventive health behavior among black and white women in urban and rural areas. *Social Science and Medicine*, 34(2), 191-198.

Eyler, A.A., Baker, E., Cromer, L., King, A.C., Brownson, R.C., Donatelle, R.J. (1998). Physical activity and minority women: A qualitative study. *Health Education and Behavior*, 25(5), 640-652.

Eyler, A.A., Brownson, R.C., Donatelle, R.J., Brown, D., Sallis, J.F. (1999). Physical activity social support and middle and older-aged minority women; results from a US survey. *Social Science and Medicine, 49*(6), 781-789.

Eyler, A.A., Matson-Koffman, D., Evenson, K., Sanderson, B., Wilbur, J., Wilcox. S., Thompson, J., Young, D. (2002). Correlates of physical activity among women from diverse racial-ethnic groups: a review. *Journal of Womens Health and Gender-Based Medicine, 11*(3), 239-253.

King, A.C., Castro, C., Wilcox S., Eyler A.A., Sallis, J.F., Brownson, R.C. (2000). Personal and environmental factors associated with physical inactivity among different racial/ethnic groups of US middle- and older-aged women. *Health Psychology, 19*(4), 354-364.

Phillips, M., Cook, J. (2001). *The 2001 Alabama State of the Heart Report.* Alabama Department of Public Health, Bureau of Health Promotion and Chronic Disease and the American Heart Association, Southeast Affiliate. Publication number ADPH-CV-1/1-01.

Sage Publications Software. (1996). *NUD*IST (Qualitative Computer Software).* Thousand Oaks, CA.

Siegel, P., Brackbill, R.M., Heath, G.W. (1995). The epidemiology of walking for exercise: implications for promoting activity among sedentary groups. *American Journal of Public Health, 85*(5), 706-710.

Wilcox, S., Castro, C., King, A.C., Housemann, R.D., Brownson, R.C. (2000). Determinants of leisure time physical activity in rural compared with urban older and ethnically diverse women in the United States. *Journal of Epidemiology and Community Health, 54*(9), 667-672.

Environmental, Policy, and Cultural Factors Related to Physical Activity in African American Women

Donna L. Richter, EdD
Sara Wilcox, PhD
Mary L. Greaney, MPH
Karla A. Henderson, PhD
Barbara E. Ainsworth, PhD

SUMMARY. Six focus groups were conducted in South Carolina with African American women (n = 42) aged 19-51 years to identify factors that influence physical activity. Transcripts were analyzed using NUD*IST.

Donna L. Richter and Mary L. Greaney are affiliated with the Department of Health Promotion, Education, and Behavior, and Sara Wilcox is affiliated with the Department of Exercise Science, Norman J. Arnold School of Public Health, University of South Carolina, Columbia, SC 29208. Karla A. Henderson is affiliated with the Department of Leisure Studies and Recreation Administration, University of North Carolina at Chapel Hill, Chapel Hill, NC 27599-3185. Barbara E. Ainsworth is affiliated with the Departments of Epidemiology and Biostatistics and Exercise Science, Norman J. Arnold School of Public Health, and Prevention Research Center, University of South Carolina, Columbia, SC 29208.

Address correspondence to: Donna L. Richter, EdD, Department of Health Promotion, Education, and Behavior, Norman J. Arnold School of Public Health, University of South Carolina, Columbia, SC 29208 (E-mail: drichter@sph.sc.edu).

The authors gratefully thank the women of Sumter County, SC, who participated in the focus groups. The authors also thank Suzette McClellan of the South Carolina Department of Health and Environmental Control for her assistance with this project. This research was supported by grant U48/CCU409664-08 from the Centers for Disease Control and Prevention.

[Haworth co-indexing entry note]: "Environmental, Policy, and Cultural Factors Related to Physical Activity in African American Women." Richter, Donna L. et al. Co-published simultaneously in *Women & Health* (The Haworth Medical Press, an imprint of The Haworth Press, Inc.) Vol. 36, No. 2, 2002, pp. 91-109; and: *Environmental, Policy, and Cultural Factors Related to Physical Activity in a Diverse Sample of Women: The Women's Cardiovascular Health Network Project* (ed: Amy A. Eyler) The Haworth Medical Press, an imprint of The Haworth Press, Inc., 2002, pp. 91-109. Single or multiple copies of this article are available for a fee from The Haworth Document Delivery Service [1-800-HAWORTH, 9:00 a.m. - 5:00 p.m. (EST). E-mail address: getinfo@haworthpressinc.com].

Cultural influences were seen as more important in determining the type of physical activity than its level. Barriers to and enablers of physical activity were identified in the social and physical environments, as were policy issues affecting physical activity in the community and at the work site. Potential community and work site interventions were suggested. Child care and monetary costs were frequently cited as barriers to physical activity. *[Article copies available for a fee from The Haworth Document Delivery Service: 1-800-HAWORTH. E-mail address: <getinfo@ haworthpressinc.com> Website: <http://www.HaworthPress.com> © 2002 by The Haworth Press, Inc. All rights reserved.]*

KEYWORDS. Physical activity, women's health, social ecology, intervention, culture, recreation, African American

PURPOSE

The purpose of the this study was to use qualitative research methods to explore cultural, environmental, and policy factors that serve as barriers or enablers to physical activity in African American women residing in the southeastern US. Qualitative methods are especially useful for generating hypotheses about groups of persons who have not been studied and who may hold beliefs that differ from the "dominant" culture (Morgan, 1998). Focus groups, a type of qualitative method, allow for the sharing of information that is most important or relevant to the group members rather than the researcher, and thus they promote the discovery of new information (Morgan, 1998). An ecological perspective of health behavior proposed by McLeroy et al. (1988) and applied to physical activity by Sallis et al. (1998) was used to conceptualize physical activity, develop the moderator's guide, and interpret our findings.

METHODS

Procedures

A representative of the local health department contacted African American women she knew were actively involved in the community (e.g., employed or active in churches or community organizations). She used a snowballing recruitment technique, asking these women to recruit other women who were in the target age group (20-50 years) and who were not engaging in regular leisure-time physical activity.

Participants were recruited from Sumter County, located in the midlands of South Carolina, approximately 45 miles east of the state capital. Rates of poverty, according to the 1990 Census (2000 data not yet available), were 20% in Sumter County, as compared to 15.4% in South Carolina and 13.1% in the U.S. (USBC, 1990). Data from the 2000 Census indicate that Sumter County's population is 104,646, with the city of Sumter being the largest city in the county (population: 39,643) (USBC, 2000). Using the rural/urban continuum codes of the U.S. Department of Agriculture, Sumter County was described in 1993 as a non-metropolitan county (UDSA, 2001). In 1993, its status changed to a metropolitan county. Thus, it is a growing county, and one that is in transition. Approximately 50% of the county's population is White, 47% is Black, and the remaining 3% of the population is from other racial/ethnic groups (USBC, 2000). The city of Sumter has a very similar racial/ethnic composition.

We conducted six focus groups, three with women aged 19-35 years (younger women) and three with women aged 36-51 years (middle-aged women). The number of participants per group ranged from five to ten, for a total of 42 women participating. Focus groups lasted 90 to 120 minutes, and were conducted in community locations familiar to the participants (i.e., community centers, a hair salon, and private homes). Focus groups were facilitated and notes were taken by experienced teams of moderators and note-takers, with each team usually including an African American woman as either moderator or note-taker. Written informed consent for focus group participation and audio-taping was obtained from all participants prior to beginning each focus group. The facilitator used an eight-question moderator's guide to elicit perceptions of what sort of policy and environmental factors were either barriers to physical activity or enablers (described in Eyler et al., 2002). Upon completion of the focus group, women were given a $20 cash incentive for participating.

Transcripts of the focus groups were prepared verbatim with names deleted. The text was then entered into QSR NUD*IST, a software program that facilitates qualitative analysis by allowing for the hierarchical coding and analysis of data across themes and groups (QSR NUD*IST, 1995). The same two USC investigators coded all transcripts, and discrepancies were resolved through discussion. Data were coded using a standardized code book developed for the Women's Cardiovascular Health Network project. The code book was arranged by domains of the ecological model (McLeroy et al., 1988; Sallis et al., 1998) to facilitate consistent coding across sites, but the sites were free to add codes unique to their populations.

Participants

A complete description of participant characteristics can be found in Eyler et al. (2002). In brief, the women were between 19 and 51 years of age, and most were single (60%), had graduated from high school (83%), and defined their health as good to excellent (85%). More than half (56%) were employed full-time or part-time. More than half (60%) reported participating in moderate activities such as brisk walking, bicycling, or vacuuming for at least 10 minutes at a time during a typical week. Thirty-two percent reported participating this often in vigorous activities such as running, aerobics, or heavy yard work.

RESULTS

Cultural Characteristics and Comparisons

Women in the focus groups were asked whether they perceived differences across cultural backgrounds in terms of women's levels of physical activity. Their responses indicated a perception that women of all cultural backgrounds are, to a great degree, "all the same" in terms of their levels of physical activity. Although women in both age ranges voiced this opinion, it came up more frequently in the middle-aged groups (ages 36 to 51 years). Examples from a middle-aged and a younger woman included:

> I don't think it has anything to do with what color, what race, or what culture you are.

> Cultural (identity) doesn't have anything (to do) with being active.

Rather than attributing differences in physical activity to cultural backgrounds, some women attributed them to individual differences, as these examples from a middle-aged and a younger woman indicate:

> It's the individual.

> I don't think that it's so much . . . the different races having different exercise values or whatever, as that some people, they're very enthusiastic about doing it.

Some women believed that cultural differences do exist. Women in the younger group said:

> It does make a difference because one culture is focused on it more so than the next culture.

> Some cultures dance. That's their way of getting physical activity. Some just plain work.

Differences in the specific leisure activities in which different cultural groups participate were noted, but these tended to be anecdotal references of a single focus group to activities that were not addressed in the other focus groups. Examples include:

Latinos dance salsa.

[Caucasian women] go to the gym.

Some sense existed among these African American women that if being physically active was associated with being lean and trim, it might not be the most desirable physical attribute. "Lots of hips and thighs" was mentioned by a younger participant as characteristic of many African American women, while Caucasian women were characterized as more focused on both appearance and health:

[Caucasian women] try to make it their business to be skinny and fit.

Some references to ethnic differences in work-related activity levels were made such as:

[Chinese] work at a faster pace.

I think those Mexicans are [more] physically active [at work] than we [African Americans] are.

Social Environmental Issues

Many social environmental factors were noted to influence how physical activity was enabled or constrained (Table 1), with social support seen as both positive and negative. Social support was referred to as support from family, friends, coworkers, community professionals, and neighbors and the roles they played in enabling or constraining physical activity, as indicated in these quotes from middle-aged women:

If you really want to get into physical activity it could be hard if you don't have anyone to help you.

If you have a group of people doing something, then I go too.

The role of family was mentioned numerous times, including the family of origin as well as the family of procreation (i.e., husband/partner and children). Several women felt that the home was a much greater influence than culture on behavior. One younger woman indicated that a person became physically active based on:

> . . . whatever you grow up with within your home . . . It's more what you get instilled in you when you're small and in bringing up . . .

Having a family member with whom one could be active was important, as were family members who acknowledged the value of physical activity. One younger woman said she was currently living with her mother, and her mother could watch her daughter so that she could take a 30-minute walk. Another told about all the household and child care help her husband gave that enabled her to have more time. A middle-aged woman described how her husband encouraged her to be active by stopping off at the Y; she said he did not mind that dinner had to be cooked later every night.

Children and other family responsibilities were perceived as both enablers and constraints. Taking care of children was seen as a type of physical activity by several women, but there seemed to be a sense among some of the younger women that it was not "enough" to make one fit. The requirements of family roles that many of the women said were central in their lives sometimes served as a barrier to physical activity. One woman said:

> The more family responsibilities you have, it's just gonna cut out as much free time as you have.

Another observed that a single parent had more opportunity for physical activity because she had to do everything [physical and otherwise] with the children as opposed to sharing the work. These comments suggest that while children were seen as interfering with planned or structured exercise, they were viewed as enablers of domestic or child care physical activity.

Friends and neighbors sometimes provided social support for physical activity. One woman said it was nice to have a friend to help encourage her to walk, and if that friend wasn't available, she tended not to walk at all instead of going on her own. One middle-aged woman suggested:

> But a co-person does help you do it more. You're more faithful.

One of the advantages of having a friend or neighbor was:

> When you're walking with somebody and you're talking, you really don't get tired.

Another woman remarked that she was the motivator for her neighborhood. When she went out to walk, others would join her. Having a neighborhood physically conducive to providing this support was also important. One middle-aged woman stated:

> . . . having a park. And having a partner.

Social support for physical activity, particularly as it pertained to recreational types of involvement, was important to these women. Families and neighborhoods were described as important potential enablers of physical activity for both younger and middle-aged participants.

Physical Environmental and Policy Issues

Women in the groups were asked to comment on how aspects of their environment, other than cultural issues and social support, constrained or enabled their physical activity. Their responses indicated that the home, work, and community environments all influenced physical activity. Both child care and the monetary costs involved in exercising applied across all these environments (Table 1).

Having a backyard or acreage around the home was cited in five of the six focus groups as an enabler. Younger women cited the backyard as a place to play active games:

> Our house is towards the highway, so we have to play in our back yard, and it's not that big but it's big enough to play kickball, tag, or freeze.

> [You can play basketball] if you got a house with a yard. Then you could get together and have little activities and things.

Having exercise equipment (treadmill, videos, and tapes) at home was mentioned occasionally as an enabler, as was the microwave oven. Having a microwave oven was perceived as minimizing the time for meal preparation, with the time saved usable for physical activity. This perception was summarized by a younger woman:

> I can throw something in the microwave, turn it on, and set my timer and go out and exercise and come back and dinner's ready.

A few women identified aspects of their household as barriers to physical activity. One younger woman noted that living in an apartment meant she did not engage in the physical activity she would get from yard work because "they handle that." Others discussed watching television:

> You tend to want to sit home, and then the TV comes on.

> Once I get in front of the TV, that's it.

TABLE 1. Factors Identified by Non-Urban African American Women as Affecting Physical Activity

Socio-Cultural	Physical Environment & Policy
<u>Social Support–As Both Enablers & Barriers</u> • Social support in general from family, friends, co-workers, neighbors • Experiences when growing up; family exposure and influence • Family members (past & current) who value physical activity • Family roles and responsibilities (e.g., child care, housework, single parenting) • Friend or neighbor to encourage or to engage in activity; "friendly neighborhood" <u>Cultural Characteristics & Comparisons</u> • Cultural influences seen as not related to level of physical activity, but to individual motivation • Cultural influences seen in type of leisure activity (e.g., salsa dance) • Cultural influences seen in work-related activity levels (e.g., work at a faster pace)	<u>Home Environment–Enablers</u> • Backyard/front yard • Exercise equipment (treadmill, videos, tapes) • Microwave (permits increased time for activity) <u>Home Environment–Barriers</u> • Apartment dwelling–lack of yard work • Watching TV <u>Work Environment–As Both Enablers & Barriers</u> • Nature of work–seated for long periods, desk job • Nature of work–active, frequent movement, lifting, walking, standing • Schedules–no time off, short and infrequent breaks, fluctuations in shifts <u>Community Environment–Barriers</u> • Heat, sun exposure • Lack of sidewalks • Traffic, fear of being hit • Lack of transportation to recreational facilities • Use of auto instead of walking <u>Community Environment–Both Enabling & Barriers</u> • Lack of community centers, facilities • Presence of parks, school facilities • Proximity of facilities, parks, neighbors–too far away • Safety–unsafe neighborhood, fear of crime, fear of dogs
<center><u>Cross-Cutting Factors: Child Care & Monetary Costs</u> • Lack of baby-sitter • Cost of joining exercise facility, gym membership</center>	

Work-related issues affecting physical activity tended to cluster around the nature of the work itself and the work schedule. The nature of the work was frequently cited by both age groups as either a barrier or an enabler. Work described as a barrier most often by middle-aged women was that requiring the woman to sit in one place for a long time. Both middle-aged and younger women described the barrier that seated work poses:

You can't just readily move as freely as you normally would in some jobs.

If you have a desk job, it's hard to exercise, because you're sitting and typing.

Some women suggested creative ways to build physical activity into jobs that require one to sit most of the time:

. . . take the elevator up and then take the stairs down.

. . . runner days . . . days when they take messages from the phone and you don't just [say] 'Hold on.' You actually take it [the message] to the next office.

Work as an enabler of physical activity was frequently cited across both age groups. A younger woman who worked in a nursing home described a typical afternoon:

When you walk in from lunch, you got to be passing out trays, feeding people. And after that you got to clean up the dining room, take all them trays out. And then . . . it's time for them to go in the bed for a nap. You got to put them down for a nap, clean them up. Then . . . you had to get them back up again.

Another younger woman, who worked in a hair salon, described her routine as equally active with constant movement "from the shampoo bowls to the dryers and back to the chair." Warehouse work, waitressing, factory work, and other jobs were described by these younger women as physically demanding, including such activities as reaching, stretching, bending, moving, walking, picking, and climbing ladders. In some jobs, it seemed that "the whole time you're there, you're exercising." Middle-aged women described some jobs as physically demanding but not as frequently as did the younger women.

Work schedules were frequently described as barriers. Having no weekends off, short lunch breaks, and shift work were all cited. One woman described the effect of a shorter lunch break:

If I can get an hour lunch break . . . with an hour I can eat the first 20 minutes and I can exercise the other 40. But 30 minutes, you really only have time to catch a snack and get back on the line.

Being too tired from long work hours also was cited as a barrier. In addition, fluctuations in work schedules that accompany swing shifts were mentioned:

> If you got one set shift and you have to do a swing shift when you got to work mornings one week and next week you got to go to work nights, that could cause you to be inactive.

Community Factors

Regarding the general physical environment in the community, heat was the barrier most frequently cited, but almost exclusively by the middle-aged groups:

> When it gets extremely hot like it is now, it's difficult to do it.

> I don't like to walk in the heat of the day.

> [Because of a skin condition] I can't be out in the sun.

Many middle-aged participants mentioned the effect of not having sidewalks on their willingness to walk in their neighborhoods, but younger women did not mention sidewalks. One middle-aged woman said of her former and current neighborhoods:

> We didn't have sidewalks, so I didn't feel comfortable walking because you never know if somebody's gonna knock you down [i.e., a vehicle would hit her]. But where I'm at right now is really nice because I have the sidewalk . . . and I've been walking, believe it or not.

Two transportation issues were cited as barriers, but only by women in the middle-aged groups. The first type was the need to access businesses or other facilities in cities or locales where they were not clustered in a small area, for example:

> [Businesses are] spread out, and you don't have transportation to get there.

> [We] don't have transportation down here. When I was in [a larger city] I [could] catch a bus anywhere.

The second transportation barrier was the forsaking of walking or biking as a means of transportation when one begins to drive a car. Middle-aged women noted:

> I kind of grew away from physical activity when I learned how to drive.

I used to walk all the way downtown before I got a car. Since I got a car, I'll drive to the store and drive downtown and get out and walk in.

Women in five of the six focus groups expressed dismay over the lack of community facilities in Sumter or the lack of "anything to do" in the community. Younger women more frequently voiced a general complaint that there was "nothing to do" in Sumter, while middle-aged women focused their comments on the lack of community facilities such as community centers or dance halls.

Women in all six focus groups agreed that parks served as enablers of physical activity in their community:

When the weather is suitable in the spring and the mild part of the fall, you can do the park thing.

[I can] walk down to the park, which is a couple of blocks [away].

Other community facilities were mentioned once, including a skating rink, a track at a church or school, the zoo, and the mall.

Proximity emerged as an enabler and lack of proximity emerged, more frequently, as a barrier. The need to drive to get to other people or to access facilities in the community was seen as a barrier for both younger and middle-aged women. A middle-aged woman noted:

If I go home, I'm not coming back. I live too far out.

Younger women noted the difficulty of getting together with friends as a deterrent to physical activity:

You have to go and meet somebody, you're getting in the car. You're driving.

I live a long way from my friends.

Several younger women put the proximity issue in perspective by observing that:

. . . if the park is close by, we can walk . . . But if [the park] is on the other side of town and I don't feel like driving, we ain't going to the park today.

[People] would walk more in the city because in the country, like Sumter, everything is spread apart, even downtown.

The difference between a large city and a small city like Sumter in terms of proximity and physical activity was captured in a quote from a younger woman:

> In the city you will look at it different. You will say, why am I going to pay a dollar to catch a bus right there when I can walk? In Sumter, you got to pay that dollar or else you'll be walking for miles. But in the city you can say, well, I'm not gonna pay no dollar when I can walk right there. You'll walk.

Proximity as an enabler was expressed by a few women, who noted that walking or riding a bike to a store was sometimes possible if the store was "not too far."

Safety concerns were frequently expressed as barriers. A general concern that the women's neighborhood was "not safe" was mentioned in four focus groups in both age groups.

> If you live in a neighborhood that's not so safe and there's always something going on, you'll be more reluctant to go out and get into physical things on the outside.

> [My neighborhood is] not really that safe. Even the policeman told us that. So, you know, I don't go any farther than the mailbox.

In addition to general concern about neighborhoods "not being safe," many specific safety issues were mentioned as barriers, with crime and unleashed or dangerous dogs mentioned most frequently. Younger women spoke of possible random violence at dance clubs rather than targeted assaults. One younger woman said:

> When you go out to a club, you just have to be careful what you doing because shots could be fired and a bullet don't got nobody's name on it. You could be right there having a good time and next thing you laying on the floor, so really it's a crime thing.

Middle-aged women's crime concerns were expressed in quotes such as:

> I just found out that one of my neighbors got raped, and I didn't even know it until someone told me.

> I just pulled up in the yard coming from the grocery store and a guy walked in our yard and came up to my car and asked me if my husband was away. I said "yeah," and he told me, "I could have you."

Unleashed or dangerous dogs were perceived as a barrier to physical activity only by women in the middle-aged groups, who did not even trust fences to provide adequate protection from dogs:

> I just get scared sometimes dogs might come out the fence.

> My next-door neighbor has a fence, but he has those Rotweilers that can jump the fence.

The comment of one middle-aged woman aptly summarized the way concerns about criminals and dogs can impinge on physical activity:

> You just want to make sure when you walk you get home safe and not be fighting off the two-legged dogs and the four-legged ones.

Cross-Cutting Issues: Child Care and Monetary Costs

The provision of child care was mentioned frequently as an enabler of physical activity, almost always by women in the younger groups. One younger woman stated:

> Can't walk today. I don't have a babysitter.

The provision of activities for children such as basketball or volleyball at adult exercise facilities was suggested. One woman explained the appeal of such an approach:

> It's more like a family thing where you don't have to go out and ask someone to baby-sit for you. Where you can just go to that one place, and everything is done at that one place.

The cost of joining an exercise facility was raised in five of the six focus groups. Middle-aged women voiced the issue succinctly:

> Who can afford it? You have to have money to exercise.

> I dropped out. I quit because I was paying more than I was getting out of it.

The cost of membership in an exercise facility is one reason that free or low-cost on-site facilities at the work site and providing reduced fees for company employees at off-site facilities were so appealing to the participants.

Intervention Suggestions

When asked to suggest interventions that would make it easier for women in their community to engage in physical activity, participants made suggestions that covered a range of interventions in the community and at the work site (Table 2).

Suggested community interventions focused on offering a variety of programs, creating facilities that enable physical activity, lowering or removing cost barriers, addressing transportation barriers, and providing child care. Among particular programs discussed, walking was the most frequently suggested, with fitness or exercise programs, team sports such as bowling or baseball, bike-a-thons, and swimming or boating also mentioned.

Recreational centers or gyms were recommended in four groups. Emphasis was placed on making them low in cost or free and on making them accessible by providing transportation, with the goal of making the centers available to all who wished to access them. The removal of cost barriers was mentioned in half the groups. Suggestions encompassed eliminating or drastically reducing gym fees ("If not free, minimal cost."), offering a sliding scale of fees ("What can you afford to pay?"), and increasing salaries ("Give them more money.") so that people do not have to work multiple jobs.

Providing transportation was proposed as a way to remove identified transportation barriers such as insufficient bus routes and the lack of other public transportation. The suggested mode of transportation in connection with the intervention was an activity bus.

The provision of child care was mentioned as an important component of the intervention in half the groups. Day care as a general enabler of physical activity was expressed by a middle-aged participant, who said:

> I would build a day care center that they could put their kids in, and then I know that if the parents had a place to send their children where they could get out to do the things that they need, then that would take a lot of the pressure off them.

Another suggested way that child care can enable physical activity was through providing this service at the exercise facility.

Interventions to address safety concerns were mentioned in two groups with specific interventions including the establishment of "crime watch" areas in neighborhoods and increasing the presence of security guards at public parks.

Suggestions for work site interventions included providing exercise facilities, schedule and break flexibility, incentives for exercising, and child care. Four groups suggested an exercise facility at the work site, which was seen as

TABLE 2. Suggested Interventions to Increase Physical Activity Among Non-Urban African American Women

Socio-Cultural	Physical	Policy
Offer programs • walking • fitness/exercise • team sports (bowling, baseball) • walk-a-thon, bike-a-thon • swimming • boating Address safety concerns • create "crime watch" areas in neighborhoods	Provide facilities • at work site • off-site with free or reduced fees for employees • in community (recreation centers, gyms)	Provide child care • more child care centers in the community • child care at exercise facilities in community • provide activities for children at exercise • facilities for adults Provide workload and schedule flexibility • reduce work load/hire more workers • rotate physically demanding jobs • longer lunch breaks • weekends off Remove/reduce cost barriers • removal of gym/recreation center fees • reduction of gym/recreation center fees • sliding scale for gym/recreation center fees • increase workers' salaries Provide incentives • movie tickets for employees who exercise • time off from work with pay to exercise Address safety concerns • more security guards in public parks

making exercise convenient for employees, especially those juggling family and work responsibilities:

> I bet more would use the gym at work, because when they have worked all day and get home and they have a family, they won't have time to really go out to a gym. If it's there for them at work, they can go into the gym at work, so that would encourage them to go ahead onto the gym. After they've done their job, they've got time to do it, they'll do it.

If a gym on-site was not possible, the women felt that proving gym memberships off-site either free or at a discount would still serve as an enabler of physical activity.

Flexibility in schedules and breaks was suggested in four focus groups as a way to increase employees' physical activity. A younger woman suggested hiring sufficient employees so that no employee had to work to exhaustion. One middle-aged woman suggested rotating jobs so that one employee was not required to always perform a particularly physically taxing duty while another had an easier task. Lunch breaks were seen as a good time for employees to "do some workout[s]," provided the breaks were long enough to allow time for physical activity as well as eating. Routinely having weekends off was mentioned as another worksite policy that would promote physical activity.

Providing incentives for participation in physical activity was suggested in four groups; incentives were seen as a way for the company to give something back to the employee and as "something that would motivate you." Specific incentives included reduced membership fees for company employees at an off-site gym, providing movie tickets to recognize those who were exercising, and paying employees while they were exercising away from work during regular work hours.

Limitations

The current study results are based on qualitative methodology using a nonrandom sample of African American women residing in the southeastern United States. Despite the best efforts of experienced moderators, some participants no doubt spoke more than others, and the views of the more vocal women may have influenced those of other participants. Since this study involved a relatively small number of African American women residing in one county of a southeastern state, their views may have limited generalizability.

DISCUSSION

Cultural Issues

Addressing questions about cultural influence is a difficult endeavor, in part because there is a close relationship between societal norms (e.g., acceptance of a larger body size) and institutional barriers (e.g., poorer access to exercise facilities and low fat foods) that influence personal behavior. Furthermore, culture is an area that is often not consciously considered when people talk about their behavior. The women in these focus groups did not attribute differences in physical activity levels to cultural background, but they did cite numerous examples of differences between cultural or ethnic groups in the specific types of leisure activities in which they engaged and in their work-related activity levels. They also felt that differences in physical activity were closely tied to individual motivation rather than cultural influences. Clearly, the role of race and ethnicity in influencing physical activity is a difficult issue to summarize. Moreover, the intersection between culture and personal situations is complicated, and it is difficult to draw meaningful conclusions and recommendations. Further exploration of the potential impact that race and ethnicity may have is needed, perhaps through a larger-scale study using both qualitative and quantitative methods

Social Environment

We found that social support played a very important role in either constraining or enabling physical activity. The presence of social support from a variety of sources (family, friends, coworkers, and neighbors) helped these women incorporate physical activity in their daily lives, while its absence constrained their physical activity. Two items frequently mentioned in this context, caring for children and having an exercise partner, offer significant insight into the design of interventions for these women. Child care acted as a constraint to structured and planned physical activities, but it served as an enabler of domestic physical activity, which is consistent with work by Sternfeld and colleagues (Sternfeld, Ainsworth, & Quesenberry, 1999). Certainly, interventions must address assistance with child care, either by providing it directly or by devising ways to incorporate physical activity into everyday interactions with children as a part of routine caregiving. Interventions should also suggest methods for incorporating exercise partners into women's daily routines, recognizing that this requires the coordination of two busy schedules.

Physical Environment and Policy

In the home environment, opportunities for intervention include time management and the provision of alternatives to watching television as recreation. Women in this study understood the value of time-saving devices such as the microwave oven and realized that such equipment can create time for physical activity in their lives. Since having a tidy home was identified in the focus groups as a cultural value for African American women, identifying opportunities for restructuring housework to either incorporate physical activity or create time for leisure activity may be beneficial. The lure of television was evident and can not be underestimated as a constraining factor. Rather than trying to motivate these women to stop watching television, interventions could include ways to be active while they were watching their favorite shows.

The aspects of the work environment most conducive to modifications to increase physical activity involved work schedules and breaks and the provision of exercise facilities for employees. These women saw the opportunity to incorporate physical activity in their lives through the workplace as perhaps their best option, but also the one over which they had the least control. Employers either provide opportunities or they do not, and in a smaller community employment options are limited. Interventions delivered at the work site would be especially appealing to these women, particularly if they are free and if child care is provided, but vouchers or discounts to exercise at nearby facilities were also appealing.

Living in a smaller community such as Sumter provided more challenges than benefits to these women in terms of their physical activity levels. Lack of transportation options and the physical layout of the community combined to make access to facilities such as parks and community recreation centers difficult. Walking to stores or facilities was not an option because of the distances involved and was made worse by a lack of sidewalks. Increasing public transportation options and providing recreational facilities in the community are essential to these women's ability to increase their physical activity.

This study's focus on environmental and policy factors that may constrain or enable physical activity contributes to an area of study that is of considerable interest to researchers but of which little is known. We should note, however, that using women's perceived barriers and enablers to physical activity to guide interventions may not translate into real behavior change. For example, although women in our groups strongly believed that work site facilities would increase their level of physical activity, a recent review reported small or no significant effect of worksite programs on fitness or physical activity levels (Dishman, Oldenburg, O'Neal, & Shephard, 1998), and other reviews have shown that work site programs tend to attract Caucasian middle-class men who are already active (Sallis & Owen, 1999). Nonetheless, our study highlights several factors that African American women view as important to their lives, and interventions that consider these factors and include members of the target community in the planning stages are more likely to succeed.

CONCLUSION

We examined cultural, environmental, and policy factors that serve as barriers to or enablers of physical activity for African American women residing in the southeastern U.S. Women easily identified how the social and physical environments influence their participation in physical activity. Social support was identified as an important enabler of physical activity, while child care responsibilities had a more complex relationship with activity: they enabled domestic activity but constrained structured activities. The non-urban environment was generally described as limiting options for physical activity. Women had relatively more difficulty articulating the role of culture, race, and ethnicity on physical activity.

REFERENCES

Dishman, R. K., Oldenburg, B., O'Neal, H., & Shephard, R. J. (1998). Worksite physical activity interventions. *American Journal of Preventive Medicine*, *15*(4), 344-361.

Eyler, A. A., Matson-Koffman, D., Vest, J. R., Evenson, K. R., Sanderson, B., Thompson, J. L., Wilbur, J., Wilcox, S., & Young, D. R. (2002). Environmental, policy, and cultural factors related to physical activity in a diverse sample of women: The Women's Cardiovascular Health Network Project–introduction and methodology. *Women & Health*, *36*(2), 1-15.

McLeroy, K. R., Bibeau, D., Steckler, A., & Glanz, K. (1988). An ecological perspective on health promotion programs. *Health Education Quarterly*, *15*(4), 351-377.

Morgan, D. L. (1998). *The focus group guidebook* (Vol. 1). Thousand Oaks, CA: Sage.

QSR NUD*IST 4 User's Guide (1995). Victoria, Australia: Qualitative Solutions and Research.

Sallis, J. F., Bauman, A., & Pratt, M. (1998). Environmental and policy interventions to promote physical activity. *American Journal of Preventive Medicine*, *15*(4), 379-397.

Sallis, J. F., & Owen, N. (1999). Interventions to promote physical activity in communities and populations, *Physical Activity and Behavioral Medicine* (pp. 153-174). Thousand Oaks, CA: Sage.

Sternfeld, B., Ainsworth, B. E., & Quesenberry, C. P. (1999). Physical activity patterns in a diverse population of women. *Preventive Medicine*, *28*(3), 313-323.

USBC. (1990) Census of Population and Housing Summary Tape 3A, South Carolina. Washington, DC: Department of Commerce, Bureau of the Census, Data User Service.

USBC. (2000). *Profile of General Demographic Characteristics, Census 2000 Summary File 1*. U.S. Census Bureau. Available: http://factfinder.census.gov [2001, September 25].

USDA. (2001). *Rural/Urban Continuum Codes*. Economic Research Service, United States Department of Agriculture. http://usda.mannli.cornell.edu/data-sets/rural/, access date 9-24-2001.

Yurgalevitch, S. M., Kriska, A. M., Welty, T. K., Go, O., Robbins, D. C., & Howard, B. V. (1998). Physical activity and lipids and lipoproteins in American Indians ages 45-74. *Medicine and Science in Sports and Exercise*, *30*(4), 543-549.

Environmental and Policy Factors Related to Physical Activity in Rural White Women

Amy A. Eyler, PhD

Joshua R. Vest, MPH

SUMMARY. Physical activity is an important aspect of health promotion and disease prevention. However, women often have lower rates of physical activity than men. The purpose of this study was to identify environmental and policy determinants to physical activity among rural white women. Six focus groups were conducted with women aged 20-50 years who were not currently regular exercisers. Women reported that the social environment had a strong impact on physical activity level. Factors of the social environment included guilt, family responsibility, and social support. Environmental and policy barriers such as lack of access to places to exercise and safety concerns were also discussed. Intervention suggestions included family exercise and work-site programs.

Amy A. Eyler and Joshua R. Vest are affiliated with Saint Louis University, School of Public Health, Prevention Research Center, St. Louis, MO.

Address correspondence to: Amy A. Eyler, PhD, Saint Louis University, School of Public Health, Prevention Research Center, 3545 Lafayette Avenue, St. Louis, MO 63104 (E-mail: eyleras@accessus.net).

The authors would like to especially thank the moderators Ann Farrell, Imogene Wiggs, Lori Dowding and Kathleen Laboray for their hard work and for letting the authors into their communities to do the research.

This research was funded through Special Interest Project 5-99 from the Centers for Disease Control and Prevention.

[Haworth co-indexing entry note]: "Environmental and Policy Factors Related to Physical Activity in Rural White Women." Eyler, Amy A. and Joshua R. Vest. Co-published simultaneously in *Women & Health* (The Haworth Medical Press, an imprint of The Haworth Press, Inc.) Vol. 36, No. 2, 2002, pp. 111-121; and: *Environmental, Policy, and Cultural Factors Related to Physical Activity in a Diverse Sample of Women: The Women's Cardiovascular Health Network Project* (ed: Amy A. Eyler) The Haworth Medical Press, an imprint of The Haworth Press, Inc., 2002, pp. 111-121. Single or multiple copies of this article are available for a fee from The Haworth Document Delivery Service [1-800-HAWORTH, 9:00 a.m. - 5:00 p.m. (EST). E-mail address: getinfo@haworthpressinc.com].

Information gained from this study can be used to fuel further research and inform future physical activity interventions. *[Article copies available for a fee from The Haworth Document Delivery Service: 1-800-HAWORTH. E-mail address: <getinfo@haworthpressinc.com> Website: <http://www. HaworthPress.com> © 2002 by The Haworth Press, Inc. All rights reserved.]*

KEYWORDS. Environment, physical activity, women's health, rural, exercise

PURPOSE

The majority of women in the United States are not optimally physically active (Macera & Pratt, 2001). In order to identify possible reasons for this inactivity, the purpose of the present study was to identify environmental and policy correlates to physical activity among white women, age 20-50 years, residing in three midwestern rural communities. The information obtained can be used to fuel further research and inform future physical activity interventions in rural areas.

METHODS

A total of six focus groups were held in three different rural communities. Two communities were in southern Missouri and one was in western Illinois. The communities were selected based on the criteria of a rural community (US Census Bureau, 2000), distance from St. Louis and other large cities, and the presence of a local contact person. Recruitment approaches included newspaper and radio advertisements, flyers which were posted by local merchants and distributed to community groups, and working with churches. In one community, flyers were sent home with all elementary school children. Having a local contact person spread the word was another approach. Recruitment flyers included a toll-free number for interested women to call for more information. All potential participants were administered a series of screening questions during the telephone call to determine eligibility. To be eligible the respondent had to be a women age 20 to 50 years, a resident of the county where the focus group was being conducted, white, and not currently a regular exerciser (moderate exercise for at least 20 minutes at a time, at least 3 times a week). The focus groups were conducted from May until August 2000. At each of the three locations, a local contact (someone living within the community being studied and who helped promote our research) was trained as the moderator. This moderator was a woman who also met the same requirements as the participants. Each session lasted from 45-60 minutes and was tape-recorded, and a research assistant was present to take notes. A demographic questionnaire was administered to all participants before the completion of the session and the women were compensated $20 for their time. The transcripts from the focus groups were analyzed using QSR NUD*IST qualitative software.

Of the 60 women who called the toll-free number, 48 were eligible and 33 actually participated. One group had only three participants, and the others ranged from four to eight. The mean age was 37 years and 79% were married. Most women (60%) were employed either full or part time and 40% said their typical workday consists of half sitting/standing and half walking. Almost 50% had some college education. Nearly all (81%) described themselves as in good (or better) health. The mean Body Mass Index calculated using self-reported height and weight was 27.8.

Recruitment for this project was difficult. Despite the varied and intense methods used and a financial incentive, interest in participating was minimal. Three of the planned groups were cancelled because of lack of interest, and in those groups that were held, many women who signed up did not show up.

RESULTS

Correlates of physical activity identified by the focus groups included the social environment, guilt and family responsibility, social support, and environmental and policy barriers (Table 1). In each focus group however, the participants did not equate "physically active" with exercising. For them, being "busy" generally meant being physically active. Most women knew they did not "exercise enough" but thought they were "active" enough.

> Hey, I feel like I am active. I might not be jogging and lifting weights, but I'll tell you I'm busy all the time.

> You'd think we'd all be skinny as rails as much as we run.

> But just constantly running all the time. Something to do with your kids, your husband. Cleaning the house. I mean to me that's gotta be some exercise somewhere in there. I'm still fat but it's gotta do something.

Social Environment

The prevailing theme of all the focus groups was the social environment. Other people, whether spouses, family members, friends, or coworkers, had significant influence on the participants' physical activity levels.

Spouses and family members were both good and bad influences with regard to physical activity. On one hand, they were described as supportive or

TABLE 1. Factors Identified by White Women that Relate to Physical Activity

Social Environment	Physical Environment & Policy
Social-Support (friends) • partners to exercise with • make exercise more social Social-Support (family) • spouses–some were supportive, others not • women needed more tangible support from spouses (help with family responsibilities) • other family members like children were supportive and served as physically active examples by being involved with sports Guilt/Family Responsibility • women felt they already had too many things to do • family responsibilities prevent time for exercise • guilt for taking time for self was prominent	Physical Environment • no sidewalks • uneven pavement • gravel roads • lived on rural highways with truck traffic Rural Area • fewer opportunities to be physically active • places too far to travel • unacceptable places to exercise (e.g., men's only bodybuilding gym) Safety • no lighting • fearful for personal safety when out walking for exercise alone Employment • working leaves no time or energy for leisure-time physical activity

good role models. For example, many had children involved with sports who kept very active or had husbands who were regular exercisers. Even when spouses or family members were not physically active, some women mentioned they supported efforts to get healthy.

> See, he wanted me to lose weight so he helped.

> Basically, what I do in life right now is my husband eats out for lunch and I hardly ever cook supper.

> I'll walk with my husband and I'll say we oughta do this more often.

Conversely, in some aspects, family members, spouses in particular, were not supportive and hindered the women's ability to take time for themselves and exercise.

> My husband laughs at me

> My husband would never go for that (referring to previous comment about not cooking supper to take time to exercise).

Guilt and Family Responsibility

Although some women mentioned that caring for children or grandchildren might increase the physical activity level, care taking and family responsibilities were the most-often mentioned reason for not taking the time to exercise. Guilt was mentioned in every one of the focus groups; women felt guilty about doing something for themselves because they had multiple roles as mother, wife, employee, caregiver, and so forth.

> I feel kind of guilty sometimes because it's just me and my son right now and we do a lot of things together like fishing and stuff like that. And I would like–if I separated us and went off and exercised, I'd feel like–I guess I was taking away time that we could be together

> I feel like a big part of our role is to respond to someone else's needs. I mean think about your own mom, you know? You were glad she was there for you and looking out for you and doing things for you. That might be why it's hard for us as women to regularly do kind of stuff (exercise) you know–have this feeling that we need to be available for everyone else.

> See part of it for me is to think that time–sometimes the time I am taking to do something–like biking or something like that, is time just for me. And then I feel guilty that I'm just using time for me.

> We give everything as well as taking care of everyone and you know, it's really–you almost feel selfish when you take time out for yourself.

The women believed that taking time to exercise was like taking time away from their family responsibilities. The only times many women felt they had "to themselves" were very early in the morning before their day started or in the evening after the kids were in bed and chores completed. These women believed they had no leisure time, and if they finally had some time to themselves at the end of the day, they would much rather watch TV or read to relax and gear up for the next day's demanding schedule.

Some of the women tried to exercise with their children (e.g., taking a walk with young children in the stroller, exercising with a video at home), but still felt the time could have been better spent on something "more productive." One woman noted that she couldn't concentrate on doing an exercise video at home when there was a pile of laundry to be done.

> And if you exercise you got 10,000 things going through your mind you should be doing instead.

In addition to the mental strain of what women "should be" doing with their time, constant demands from others had a serious impact on women's intention to exercise.

It's like, "Mom! Mom!" I mean there's no time for yourself unless you get up and make the time. And who wants to get up at 4:30 in the morning and work out?

It's one more thing. It's like going to get groceries. It's like mowing the grass. It's like one more thing to have to do.

Social Support

Another aspect of the social environment that was mentioned in all the focus groups was social support. Most women mentioned that exercising would be easier if they had a partner or someone who would hold them accountable. Exercising with someone made time go by faster and made exercise seem less like a chore. Also, the women reported that a friend or someone to exercise with could be a major motivating factor in maintaining a program.

When you get out there and you're with someone, before you know it, the hour's up. But when you are by yourself, you are thinking "What time is it?"

If I had someone calling me saying "You gonna do it? You gonna do it?" And I'm like yeah, I guess I'm gonna do it.

Environmental and Policy Barriers

Living in a Rural Area

Women in all the groups believed they had fewer opportunities for exercise because they lived in a rural area. Exercise facilities were few and not close to most of their homes. Some communities did have a gym or exercise facility, but the women perceived them as being geared toward men. Women in all groups were adamant about the need for a "women's only" place to exercise. In fact, a well-marketed franchise of "women's-only" toning/exercise facilities was requested by participants in every single focus group.

I'd feel more comfortable at a place just for women. You would feel a lot more comfortable than walking around a track with 75 idiots out there playing ball going "hey."

I'd go to a Curves for Women. It's guaranteed to work and it doesn't cost a whole lot to join. And it's only women.

The participants all knew of places in nearby larger towns where they had community centers or exercise programs, but it wasn't feasible to travel that far on a daily, or even weekly, basis.

> There's no way we could just travel 45 minutes to Poplar Bluff to exercise. I just don't have time in my day.

> They have a nice community center up there. It's just too far away from where I live.

In addition to lack of facilities, a major complaint of women was lack of sidewalks. Walking seemed to be the activity that most of the women were willing to do for exercise, but lack of sidewalks hindered them. Uneven pavement and traffic were cited as problems. Many women lived on gravel roads or two-lane highways without sidewalks.

> I mean I don't live right in town and there's no sidewalks. If you're in town, there's sidewalks and you see people walking in town all the time, but boy, you never see that here, you'd get run over!

> I wouldn't walk on our road. No way. Poor Vicki has ended up in the ditch walking on that road!

Personal safety was a concern in most groups. Poor lighting at night and people "hanging around" were deterrents to outdoor physical activities. Having an exercise partner or a husband who would walk with them were discussed as an option to overcome these barriers.

Policy Factors

The majority of the women were employed outside the home. Some had physically demanding jobs such as heavy commercial kitchen work or health care positions that required lifting and carrying. Others had sedentary jobs (bus driver, teacher, phone sales). Exercising at work was one option for incorporating more exercise and most of the women thought they could be more physically active if their work schedules were more flexible. Many participants cited long hours and very long days. Exercising before or after work would not be feasible because of caregiving responsibilities. Suggestions for work-site interventions included onsite exercise facilities or time off work to exercise.

> Hey if everyone will exercise instead of working till five, you can work until four!

> You come with me and exercise, and I'll give you a longer lunch hour.

A place to exercise would be nice, where I used to work, they had a gym right in the facility and so on your lunch break or after work or before work you could work out. It was very convenient.

As one women noted, however, the mere presence of facilities or time off would not be enough. "They could pay me to do it!" was her comment.

Intervention Suggestions

Most of the intervention suggestions involved building places for exercise that did not cost a lot to use, having separate facilities for women, and having programs for children (see Table 2). Additional suggestions were to improve sidewalks and lighting and make it safer to exercise outdoors. Participants also cited the work-site and churches as potential places for exercise interventions.

Most of the women agreed that just having a place to exercise would not be enough and they described two potential motivating factors to enhance participation in exercise. One was social support from family members and friends, which was recommended for both motivation to begin and maintain an exercise program. The second factor was support from spouses or family members, which was suggested in two ways. First, husbands or children could actually do the activities with the women; for example, husbands could walk with them or their children could participate in concurrent sporting or exercise programs. Second, family members and spouses could support the women in other ways, such as being flexible in their expectations of cooking, cleaning, etc.

In addition to social support, financial incentives were suggested. It was clear that this group of women did not want to spend a lot of money to exercise. Financial incentives recommended were low-cost programs, discounts on insurance rates, and monetary prizes for participation.

TABLE 2. Physical Activity Intervention Suggestions from Rural White Women

Social	Physical	Policy
• Helps others motivate • Organize team sports for women only • Build support network • Buddy-system	• Pave roads • Improve sidewalks • Build walking and bicycle trails • Provide bicycle rentals • Build shopping mall for indoor walking Build a civic center that includes specialty areas, programs: • Swimming pool • Walking track • Women's only gym • Childcare center	• Provide exercise program at work • Provide flexible schedules to exercise • Provide childcare • Make program low or no-cost • Work with insurance companies to provide discount • Provide incentives and prizes for sustained motivation

DISCUSSION

Research shows that women have less leisure time than men (Henderson, Shaw, Bialeschki, & Freysinger, 1995), in part, because of work, family, and other commitments (e.g., church). The women in our study made it abundantly clear that exercising was not a priority in their lives. It was difficult to take time for themselves without feeling guilty. Although they noted the importance of exercise as part of a healthy lifestyle and believed they "should" be doing it, the women thought there was not enough time in the day to do what "needs" to be done without adding something else like exercise. This is not a new finding. Women have been socialized to put family needs first (Henderson et al., 1995) and the multiple roles as wife, mother, employee, etc., are both physically and mentally taxing. Prior research concurs with our findings (Barnekow-Bergkvist, Hedberg, Janler, & Jansson, 1996; Eyler et al., 1998; Sternfeld et al., 1999; Verhoef et al., 1992; Yoshida et al., 1988).

The second major point the women in our study made was that living in a rural area made it difficult to exercise. In particular, lack of facilities or sidewalks make it hard or inconvenient to exercise. Previous research on the impact of rural residence has yielded mixed results. In one study, King et al. (2000) found that in a large cross sectional survey of diverse women, there was no significant difference in the correlates of physical activity between rural and urban women (King et al., 2000). In contrast, analysis of the Behavioral Risk Factor Surveillance System Survey found that physical inactivity was highest in rural areas (Centers for Disease Control and Prevention, 1998). However, Brownson et al. (2000) found that access to a walking trail significantly increased walking for exercise in a rural sample of women (Brownson et al., 2000b).

A third major point was the importance of combining physical activity with an already existing responsibility (e.g., work, childcare). One place that holds promise for increasing exercise is the workplace; the women claimed they would be more likely to exercise if they could fit it in to their workday. Participants also suggested family physical activities so as not to take time away from children or spouses.

CONCLUSION

In conclusion, our findings are important for planning physical activity interventions with this population. A program or facility to increase physical activity will probably not be particularly successful by itself. Interventions should work on building support networks as well as facilities, and those networks that build on friendship and childcare may have greater effectiveness. In addition to support networks and facilities, programs need to be family oriented. Whether an intervention offers concurrent programming for children, childcare, or family activities, these factors would make this population more likely to participate because of their strong family commitment.

Focus groups such as ours are an important first step toward gaining an understanding of a unique population before planning interventions. The types of barriers reported by the women in our sample need to be addressed if interventions are to be successful.

REFERENCES

Barnekow-Bergkvist, M., Hedberg, G., Janler, U., & Jansson, E. (1996). Physical activity pattern in men and women at the ages of 16 and 34 and development of physical activity from adolescence to adulthood. *Scandinavian Journal of Medicine & Science in Sports*, *6*, 359-370.

Brownson, R.C., Eyler, A.A., King, A.C., Brown, D.R., Shyu, Y.L., & Sallis, J.F. (2000a). Patterns and correlates of physical activity among US women 40 years and older. *American Journal of Public Health*, *90*(2), 264-70.

Brownson, R.C., Housemann, R.A., Brown, D.R., Jackson-Thompson, J., King, A.C., Malone, B.R., & Sallis, J. (2000b). Promoting physical activity in rural communities; Walking trail access, use, and effects. *American Journal of Preventive Medicine*, *18*(3), 235-241.

Centers for Disease Control and Prevention. (1998). Self-reported physical inactivity by degree of urbanization–United States, 1996. *Morbidity and Mortality Weekly Report*, *47*(50), 1097-1100.

Eyler, A., Baker, E., Cromer, L., King, A., Brownson, R., & Donatelle, R. (1998). Physical activity and minority women: A qualitative study. *Health Ed Behavior*, *25*, 640-652.

Eyler, A., Brownson, R., Donatelle, R., Brown, D., & Sallis, J. (1999). Physical activity social support and middle- and older-aged minority women: Results from a US survey. *Social Science and Medicine*, *49*(6), 781-789.

Eyler, A., Wilcox, S., Matson-Koffman, D., Evenson, K., Sanderson, B., Thompson, J., Wilbur, J., & Young, D. (2002). Determinants of physical activity among women from diverse racial/ethnic groups: A review. *Journal of Women's Health and Gender-Based Medicine*, *11*(3), 239-253.

Henderson, K., Shaw, S., Bialeschki, M., & Freysinger, V. (1995). *Both Gains and Gaps*. State College, PA: Venture Publishing.

King, A. (1997). Intervention strategies and determinants of physical activity and exercise behavior in adult and older adult men and women. *World Review of Nutrition and Dietetics*, *82*, 148-158.

King, A., Castro, C., Wilcox, S., Eyler, A., Sallis, J., & Brownson, R. (2000). Personal and environmental factors associated with physical inactivity among different racial-ethnic groups of US middle-aged and older-aged women. *Health Psychology*, *19*(4), 354-364.

Macera, C.A. and M. Pratt. (2000). Public health surveillance and physical activity. *Research Quarterly for Exercise and Sport*, *71*(20), 97-103.

Sternfeld, B., Ainsworth, B.E., & Quesenberry, C.P. (1999). Physical activity patterns in a diverse population of women. *Preventive Medicine, 28*(13), 313-323.

US Department of Health and Human Services. (1996). Physical activity and health: A report of the Surgeon General. Atlanta, GA: U.S. Department of Health and Human Services, Center for Disease Control and Prevention, National Center for Chronic Disease Prevention and Health Promotion.

US Census Bureau. (2000). <http://www.census.gov/geo>.

Verhoef, M., Love, E., & Rose, M. (1992). Women's social roles and their exercise participation. *Women and Health, 19*(4), 15-28.

Yoshida, K., Allison, K., & Osborn, R. (1988). Social factors influencing perceived barriers to physical activity among women. *Canadian Journal of Public Health, 79*, 104-108.

Environmental, Policy, and Cultural Factors Related to Physical Activity in a Diverse Sample of Women: The Women's Cardiovascular Health Network Project– Summary and Discussion

Amy A. Eyler, PhD
Joshua R. Vest, MPH
Bonnie Sanderson, PhD
JoEllen Wilbur, PhD

Dyann Matson-Koffman, PhD
Kelly R. Evenson, PhD
Janice L. Thompson, PhD
Sara Wilcox, PhD

Deborah Rohm Young, PhD

Amy A. Eyler and Joshua R. Vest are affiliated with Saint Louis University, School of Public Health, Prevention Research Center, St. Louis, MO 63104. Dyann Matson-Koffman is affiliated with the Cardiovascular Health Branch, Division of Adult and Community Health, National Center for Chronic Disease Prevention and Health Promotion, CDC, Atlanta, GA 30341-3724. Kelly R. Evenson is affiliated with the University of North Carolina-Chapel Hill, School of Public Health, Department of Epidemiology, Chapel Hill, NC 27514. Bonnie Sanderson is affiliated with the University of Alabama, Birmingham, AL 35294. Janice L. Thompson is affiliated with the Department of Pediatrics, Center for Health Promotion & Disease Prevention, University of New Mexico Sciences Center, Albuquerque, NM 87131. JoEllen Wilbur is affiliated with the University of Illinois at Chicago, Department of Public Health, Mental Health, and Administrative Nursing, College of Nursing, Chicago, IL 60612-7350. Sara Wilcox is affiliated with the Department of Exercise Science, Norman J. Arnold School of Public Health, University of South Carolina, Columbia, SC 29208. Deborah Rohm Young is affiliated with Johns Hopkins University, Welch Center for Prevention, Epidemiology, and Clinical Research, Baltimore, MD 21205.

Address correspondence to: Amy A. Eyler, PhD, Saint Louis University, School of Public Health, Prevention Research Center, 3545 Lafayette Avenue, St. Louis, MO 63104 (E-mail: eyleras@accessus.net).

[Haworth co-indexing entry note]: "Environmental, Policy, and Cultural Factors Related to Physical Activity in a Diverse Sample of Women: The Women's Cardiovascular Health Network Project–Summary and Discussion." Eyler, Amy A. et al. Co-published simultaneously in *Women & Health* (The Haworth Medical Press, an imprint of The Haworth Press, Inc.) Vol. 36, No. 2, 2002, pp. 123-134; and: *Environmental, Policy, and Cultural Factors Related to Physical Activity in a Diverse Sample of Women: The Women's Cardiovascular Health Network Project* (ed: Amy A. Eyler) The Haworth Medical Press, an imprint of The Haworth Press, Inc., 2002, pp. 123-134. Single or multiple copies of this article are available for a fee from The Haworth Document Delivery Service [1-800-HAWORTH, 9:00 a.m. - 5:00 p.m. (EST). E-mail address: getinfo@haworthpressinc.com].

123

SUMMARY. Ethnic minority and low-income populations have the highest rates of cardiovascular disease and the lowest rates of leisure-time physical activity. Because physical activity reduces the risk of premature death and disability from cardiovascular disease, researching correlates to such activity in these populations is an important aspect of health promotion in the US. To identify environmental, policy, and cultural barriers to physical activity in women, The Women's Cardiovascular Health Network Project conducted focus groups with White, African American, Latina, and American Indian women aged 20-50 years. The focus groups were audiotaped, transcribed, and analyzed with QSR NUD*IST qualitative software using a set of codes developed a priori by the research team. Family priorities were a main barrier to physical activity in all the groups. Having multiple roles as wife, mother, daughter, and as an active community member was mentioned as time-consuming and difficult, leaving little time or energy for exercise. Cultural barriers, which varied among the groups, included acculturation issues, lack of community support, and lack of past experience with exercise. Physical activity interventions suggested involved work programs, family-friendly programs, increased social support, and the availability of safer places to exercise such as parks, well-lit walking trails, and recreation centers. Many of the barriers were common to all groups (e.g., family priority) while some were unique (e.g., lack of community support). Assessing and addressing the issues raised should be considered when planning physical activity interventions for these populations. *[Article copies available for a fee from The Haworth Document Delivery Service: 1-800-HAWORTH. E-mail address: <getinfo@haworthpressinc.com> Website: <http://www. HaworthPress.com> © 2002 by The Haworth Press, Inc. All rights reserved.]*

KEYWORDS. Policy, environment, physical activity, women, exercise

OVERVIEW

Physical activity is an important part of health promotion and disease prevention (USDHHS, 1996). Reducing disparities in health and increasing physical activity levels in all populations is paramount to the future health of our nation. For physical activity interventions to be effective, however, they must adequately address barriers to activity and promote factors that enable it. As indicated by our projects in this series, these barriers and enablers are both common and unique across race/ethnicity. Common barriers, such as lack of time, have been cited in previous research (Carter-Nolan, Adams-Campbell, & Williams, 1996; Eyler et al., 1998; Fischer et al., 1999; Fitzgerald, Singleton, Neale, Prasas, & Hess, 1994; Jaffee, Lutter, Rex, Hawkes, & Bucaccio, 1999;

Sternfeld, Ainsworth, & Quesenberry, 1999; USDHHS, 1996) while barriers such as lack of community support for exercise (Thompson et al., 2002) may be unique to specific populations.

In this article, we summarize the findings from this multi-site, focus group project. Introductory information and methodology for this project are reported elsewhere (Eyler et al., 2002). The findings add important information to the scarce body of literature on environmental, policy and cultural barriers to physical activity in this diverse population of women.

SUMMARY OF RESULTS

A summary of results is depicted in Table 1.

TABLE 1. Summary of Main Environmental Factors Related to Physical Activity Identified by African American, American Indian, Latina, and White Women. The Women's Cardiovascular Health Network Project, 2001

Socio-Cultural	Physical Environment & Policy
Social Support • need support from family friends, co-workers, community • need help balancing demands of multiple roles in order to make time for physical activity • identifying with role models and having motivational support would help	**Physical** • weather (e.g., heat, wind, cold) and lack of daylight were barriers • lack of sidewalks, pavement for walking • traffic makes it difficult to walk for exercise • distance to facilities too great or too difficult
Cultural Factors • physical activity not a top priority • other's (e.g., husband, community) views greatly influence physical activity level • language and acculturation issues may hinder physical activity • lack of prior experience or knowledge affects physical activity • larger body size may hinder physical activity • child care issues • need traditional dances and cultural events as a means of increasing physical activity	**Policy** • many places cost probative • need child care provision • employer-supported programs and events would be helpful • personal safety concerns (e.g., people, dogs)

General Perceptions About Lifestyles

How a woman defines physical activity is an important aspect of assessment of physical activity levels and a necessary component of an intervention. As part of the moderators' introduction to the groups, *physical activity* was defined as many things. Heavy housework, walking to the store, work or other places, bicycle riding, and swimming were given as examples of physical activity. Even though we defined physical activity as many different things, the participants spoke of exercise as something separate from day-to-day physical activities, and most considered themselves to be active but not *exercisers*. Participants said that having multiple roles of wife, mother, daughter, employee, and community member led to a "busy-ness" that they perceived as physical activity.

Although they thought of themselves as physically active, they did not think it was enough to gain health benefits. Most of the women knew of the importance of *exercising* for good health and that they "should" do it. Two of the groups (African American and American Indian) identified their past culture as being more physically active, recalling farming or other activities of past generations that made physical activity an inherent part of daily life. Participants noted, however, that factors such as sedentary jobs, motorized vehicles, and microwave ovens had replaced these physically active lifestyles. Latina women reported being more active earlier in their own lives, recalling life in their home-country where walking was the main mode of transportation.

Family and Caregiving Responsibilities

The most prominent subject of discussion across all groups was the role of family and caregiving and its effect on physical activity. All the groups indicated that their family responsibilities were a priority in their life, and that these responsibilities were time-consuming and arduous. Child care, husband-care, cooking, cleaning, yard work, and other tasks (often in addition to work responsibilities) left little spare time for these women. A few women considered themselves more physically active because of these responsibilities, but did not feel they gained any health benefit from them.

Women in several groups mentioned that because of these responsibilities, they felt selfish or guilty doing something for themselves. Single parenting, social expectations, or heavy community involvement made it difficult to justify spending time on exercise or any other form of self-care. In the Latina groups, the theme of 'familism' came through clearly, with children, husband, and household duties all having higher priority than interest in physical activity. The women placed such things before their own personal needs and prioritized their family's health over their own.

The American Indian groups mentioned that traditional physical activity such as dance or agricultural activities were accepted, but that their cultural community frowned upon women who exercised for the sole purpose of exercising (e.g., walking for exercise). These women, in particular, felt there was a great deal of social and cultural pressure to conform to their roles as mothers and caretakers. In their attempt to meet societal expectations, American Indian women reported that they are not encouraged to take care of themselves, and they find it difficult to add regular physical activity to their responsibilities (Thompson et al., 2002).

A second prominent discussion point of this project was the social environment, with social support discussed in many forms in all groups. The women mentioned that individual support from friends, family, or spouses would help motivate and support an exercise habit; friends or family members could serve as exercise partners for motivation and camaraderie, for example. More tangible support, such as help with housework or chores would free up time that could be used for exercise.

Urban African American, American Indian, and Latina women mentioned the importance of a different kind of support, that of the *community*. It was recommended that women band together in a community coalition to help each other exercise more. In the American Indian population, desired community support for physical activity took the form of the backing of tribal leaders and changing existing social norms to be more accepting of physically active women. Latina women suggested community support in another way. Because of acculturation issues and language barriers, many Latinas did not feel connected to the community. Community support would need to come in the form of enhanced communication; for example, community programs would need to disseminate information in Spanish or hold classes with bilingual instructors.

Safety Concerns

Concerns with safety, the form of which differed to some extent between rural and urban areas, were raised in all groups. Urban women were concerned about being harassed by homeless persons and drug dealers or being a victim of a drive-by shooting. Many urban women knew of places for exercise, but they had to go outside their immediate community to travel there, and they perceived doing so was unsafe. Rural women were also concerned about harassment from strangers, but they were also afraid to walk on roads without sidewalks because of uneven pavement, dust, insects, and fast-moving traffic. Both urban and rural groups mentioned fear of being attacked by unleashed or stray dogs and indicated this impeded many outdoor activities, walking in particular.

Work

Sixty-three percent of women in our sample were employed and discussions about work and how it affected physical activity were common. Three groups (rural African American, urban African American and rural White) identified themselves as hard workers and having physically demanding jobs, leaving them too tired to do much of anything after work. When asked whether their bosses or workplaces encouraged the women to exercise, one woman commented "the only thing they do is encourage us to work more."

Most of the women who worked did not have flexible hours or much of an opportunity to increase their physical activity at work. Many heard of companies that allowed time for employees to exercise and thought that was a good idea, but they doubted that it would be an option at their own jobs.

Cultural Issues

When the groups were asked to comment on perceptions of cultural differences in physical activity levels between different races/ethnicities, the responses were similar. For example, the majority of comparisons were made to white women. Most groups indicated that White women had more financial resources to be more physically active and that being thin and fit is more a part of the white culture than it is for women of color.

Participants also said that White women were "brought up" to know how to exercise and both African American and Latina women commented on their own lack of prior experience in this area. Latinas indicated that young girls were not encouraged to be as physically active as boys and this had a negative effect on physical activity levels as the girls became adult women. African American women, in turn, indicated that their role models during their childhood were too busy with caregiving responsibilities to exercise or do any type of self-care. Without role models, it was difficult to adopt physical activity themselves.

Body size and "cultural eating" were mentioned by American Indian and African American women. Both groups indicated that a heavier body weight was more acceptable in their culture than it was for White women. White women were perceived as being "obsessed with thinness." The American Indian and African American heavier body size was attributed mainly to their diets. High-fat, fried, traditional foods were cited as important parts of both cultures. African American and American Indian women mentioned that after eating a heavy meal of traditional foods, they lacked the energy to exercise.

The most common cultural comparison was in the area of family responsibility. African American, American Indian, and Latina women felt that they "bear the burden of their families" far more than White women. One women summed it up by saying, "we always do it ourselves (referring to child care and housekeeping), not hire someone to do it." Some Latina and American Indians indicated they would not put their children in child care because it was their own responsibility to watch the children and they would not trust anyone else. This obligation to family was cited as a major barrier to physical activity.

White and African American women perceived Asian women as more physically active because of their culture. Asian women were thought to have smaller bodies, do more physical labor in the home, and have healthier diets than the other groups.

Even though participants were quick to note perceived cultural differences in physical activity levels and reasons for these differences, some groups mentioned that differences in physical activity levels were not a matter of cultural differences but rather individual factors, such as lack of motivation. They said that women who really wanted to exercise would find a way despite their cultural or societal barriers.

Suggested Interventions

Table 2 summarizes the main suggested interventions from the focus group participants. All the groups suggested interventions involving children and families and prioritized the provision of childcare, more family activities, and concurrent programming for all ages.

Specific environmental and policy changes were suggested in all of the groups. Several of the policy suggestions focused on financial issues. The lack of places to walk prompted suggestions for building tracks, malls, or other places where women could do so. Participants also recommended sliding fee scales for recreation centers and fitness clubs and discounts on health insurance for exercisers. They also suggested monetary bonuses for exercising and other incentives to increase their motivation to be active.

Recommended environmental changes centered largely on safety. A need for safer places to exercise in communities was apparent in all groups. Parks, well-lit walking trails, and community recreation centers that are safe and comfortable places for women to exercise are seemingly sparse in many of the communities.

LIMITATIONS

There are several limitations of this study. First, in spite of the diversity of the sample, Asian women were not represented. Since the populations were chosen by the funding organization's assessment of grant applications and none of the applications included Asian women, this population was not researched. Asian women are greatly underrepresented in physical activity research, and future study of this population is a priority. Second, the data

TABLE 2. Summary of Physical Activity Intervention Suggestions from African American, American Indian, Latina, and White Women Participants in the Women's Cardiovascular Health Network Project, 2001

Socio-Cultural	Physical	Policy
• involve family members • organize programs in churches • provide competent instructors and role models • support groups • women-only facility • organize child care activities • conduct informational sessions • increase support of spouse and community	• build or open new facilities such as community centers, pools, walking trails • build a women-only facility • build sidewalks • eliminate escalators and elevators • pave roads • build or improve lighting in parks and on streets • build playgrounds	• provide funding for maintenance or clean up grounds of existing recreational grounds • provide transportation to and from exercise facilities • encourage employers to make flexible schedules • provide financial assistance with cost of programs • address safety concerns

collected may not be generalizable to the populations studied, particularly within ethnic minority groups that are made up of many diverse subgroups (e.g., American Indian Tribes or Latinas from different origin countries). Third, the use of focus groups to collect data has limitations similar to other self-report data collection methods whereas the information gained may be biased by the individual's perception of the situation which may or may not be comparable to a more objective assessment. Additionally, the difference in the way participants perceived physical activity by definition (i.e., by quantitative assessment) versus what their "actual" physical activity levels were, was evident. Despite these limitations, the qualitative method used here helped us gain valuable preliminary information that will inform a quantitative instrument for Phase II of our project.

DISCUSSION

These groups of women identified family responsibilities as both their principal life priority and the foremost barrier to increasing physical activity. In many cultures, women have been socialized to put family needs first (Henderson, 1995) and researchers and practitioners must consider this before they plan and implement effective interventions. Several recommendations from our study seem like viable options. For example, programs for women that occur at the same time and place as programs for family members, or more family-friendly activities, seem to be a welcomed alternative to women taking time out of their busy schedules "just" to exercise. A practical solution would be a playground for children surrounded by a walking track. The women could walk for exercise while their children played.

Environmental and policy changes are necessary if interventions are to be successful. Work site policies can aid in increasing physical activity levels. Because many of these women have family responsibilities after work, it makes sense to incorporate physical activity into their work day. The women suggested flexible hours, onsite facilities, and extra time off to exercise. We should consider, however, that even though the women in our study say that these changes would help them increase their exercise, research shows that only about 20-30% of the eligible population actually participate in employee fitness programs (Dishman, 1998). Programs should assess unique barriers and interests of the employed, non-professional women in order to design effective programs (e.g., desire not to sweat, women-only programs).

Environmental and policy changes can also improve safety, another major barrier. Making such changes is a major undertaking, however, with financial resources and community support needed as key elements of success. Additionally, facilities must include resources that address other barriers to physical activity, such as child care or cost.

CONCLUSION AND RECOMMENDATIONS

From this research we have learned that increasing physical activity levels of women may be a challenging task, especially in minority populations. Barriers need to be assessed and addressed if interventions are to be successful. Based on our findings, we have developed five practical recommendations:

Finding 1: Family responsibilities are the number one priority for the majority of these women.

Recommendation: Physical activity interventions must address this strong feeling when planning community-based programs or building facilities. This may include providing child care alternatives or promoting family-inclusive physical activity programs.

Finding 2: The social environment is a strong influence on physical activity among women.

Recommendation: Enhancing the social support systems within community-based and worksite interventions should be an integral part of physical activity promotion among women.

Finding 3:   Many populations have unique cultural or perceived barriers to physical activity.

Recommendation: Finding ways of making activities culturally-relevant to women (e.g., through traditional dance) is recommended. These barriers need to be assessed and incorporated into program planning and implementation and are likely accomplished by having representative community members involved in the process, particularly women.

Finding 4:   Environmental and policy issues are perceived as barriers to physical activity among women.

Recommendation: Communities, institutions, and governmental agencies must assess their existing environment and policies to identify opportunities for improvement that may impact physical activity behaviors, especially in women. For example, policy may procure funding for enhancement (e.g., lighting, maintenance) of walking trails or tracks in the community.

Finding 5:   Policy changes must be considered at multiple levels–home, neighborhood, worksite, community, and government, to promote sustainable environments for physical activity for women.

Recommendation: Policy changes must go beyond increasing access to facilities or programs and incorporate ways to build ongoing and effective support for physical activity in the community. It is evident from our findings that in addition to environmental and policy factors, personal, social, and cultural factors play a role in increasing physical activity in women. Merely building an exercise facility may not help women in these communities become more active. Developing and maintaining positive and culturally appropriate physical activity messages and support systems may be just as important as access.

In summary, women in this study made recommendations for physical activity interventions that address multiple areas–the family, social and cultural issues, the physical environment, and policy (see Figure 1). This suggests that a more integrated approach may be needed to increase physical activity among diverse racial and ethnic populations.

FIGURE 1. A model of an integrated approach to increasing physical activity among ethnic/minority populations of women.

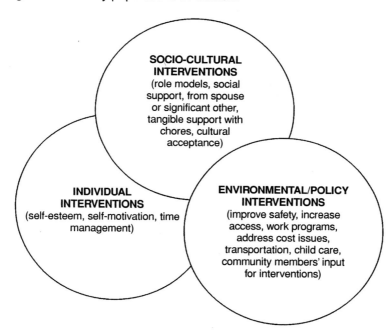

REFERENCES

Carter-Nolan, P.L., Adams-Campbell, L.L., & Williams, J. (1996). Recruitment strategies for black women at risk for noninsulin-dependent diabetes mellitus into exercise protocols: a qualitative assessment. *Journal of the National Medical Association, 88*(9), 558-562.

Eyler, A.A., Baker, E., Cromer, L., King, A.C., Brownson, R.C., & Donatelle, R.J. (1998). Physical activity and minority women: A qualitative study. *Health Education and Behavior, 25*, 640-652.

Eyler, A.A., Matson-Koffman, D., Vest, J.R., Evenson, K.R., Sanderson, B., Thompson, J.L., Wilbur, J., Wilcox, S., & Young, D.R. (2002). Environmental, policy, and cultural factors related to physical activity in a diverse sample of women: The Women's Cardiovascular Health Network Project–introduction and methodology. *Women & Health, 36*(2), 1-15.

Fischer, I., Brown, D., Blanton, C., Casper, M., Croft, J., & Brownson, R. (1999). Physical activity patterns of Chippewa and Menominee Indians: The Inter-Tribal Heart Project. *American Journal of Preventive Medicine, 17*(3), 189-197.

Fitzgerald, J., Singleton, S., Neale, A., Prasas, A., & Hess, J. (1994). Activity levels, fitness status, exercise knowledge, and exercise beliefs among healthy, older African American and White women. *Journal of Aging and Health, 6*(3), 297-312.

Jaffee, L., Lutter, J.M., Rex, J., Hawkes, C., & Bucaccio, P. (1999). Incentives and barriers to physical activity for working women. *American Journal of Health Promotion, 13*(4), 215-218, iii.

Sternfeld, B., Ainsworth, B.E., & Quesenberry, C.P. (1999). Physical activity patterns in a diverse population of women. *Preventive Medicine, 28*(13), 313-323.

Thompson, J.L., Allen, P., Cunningham-Sabo, L., Yazzie, D.A., Curtis, M., & Davis, S.M. (2002). Environmental, policy, and cultural factors related to physical activity in sedentary American Indian women. *Women & Health, 36*(2), 59-74.

United States Department of Health and Human Services. (1996). Physical Activity and Health: A Report of the Surgeon General. Atlanta, GA: U.S. Department of Health and Human Services, Center for Disease Control and Prevention, National Center for Chronic Disease Prevention and Health Promotion.

Index

African American women
    rural, 75-90. *See also* Rural African
    American women
    South Carolina study, 91-109. *See*
    also South Carolina study
African American women
    urban, 17-28. *See also* Urban
    African American women
    urban well-educated, 29-41. *See*
    also Urban well-educated
    African American women
(University of) Alabama–Birmingham,
    75-90
American Indian women: sedentary,
    59-74
    conclusions, 72-73
    discussion, 69-72
    environmental and policy issues,
    67-69
    interventions suggested, 69
    methods, 61-62
    purpose of study, 60-61
    results, 62-69
    sociocultural issues, 62-67

Behavioral Risk Factor Surveillance
    System (BRFSS), 2,3-4
Body image, 83
Body size preferences, 36-37

Caregiving responsibilities, 126-127
Centers for Disease Control and
    Prevention (CDC), 4
Community, as defined by study, 7

Community factors, African American
    women: South Carolina
    study, 100-103
Conclusion and recommendations,
    131-133
Cultural factors
    African American women: rural,
    82-84
    African American women: South
    Carolina study, 94-95
    African American women: urban,
    21-22
    in physical activity, 3
    summary and conclusions, 128-129
    urban well-educated African
    American women, 35-37
Cultural responsibilities, 36-37
Culture, as defined by study, 8

Demographics, of focus groups, 9-10

Employment concerns, 128
Environment, as defined by study, 7
Environmental factors
    African American women: urban,
    22-23
    American Indian women, 67-69
    Latina immigrant women, 46-48

Family, role of, 31-32
Family responsibilities, 126-127
Family support, 48-49
Focus group questions, 6